Herbs:
The Magic Healers

Herbs:
The Magic Healers

Paul Twitchell

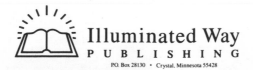

Illuminated Way
PUBLISHING
P.O. Box 28130 • Crystal, Minnesota 55428

Herbs:
The Magic Healers

This book does not propose to replace the services of anyone's family physician, who should be consulted for conditions requiring his services.

Cover design by
Stan Burgess and Phil Morimitsu
Second edition—1986
Third printing—1988

This special edition has been updated by A. Stuart Wheelwright, master herbalist, nutritionist, and biochemist.

Contents

Foreword

The ancient lore of herbs and their magic healing properties comes alive in these pages, as Paul Twitchell — modern-day founder of Eckankar, the Ancient Science of Soul Travel — reveals the ancient message of spiritual freedom to all who long for greater physical, emotional, mental, and spiritual well-being.

Since the earliest history of life on this planet, herbs have been used by health practitioners and spiritual adepts alike for their remarkable healing properties. Today, after a brief detour into inorganic medicines, mankind is again being directed to the proper use of herbs — God's medicines — to restore to abundant health a disease-ridden world.

This book brings new insights into the ancient herbal lore long hidden in remote corners of the world and new horizons for those in anguish of body and Soul. It lets each individual discover his own innate viewpoint (Soul's view) and how to apply it to the healing magic locked in herbs and nutrition.

There is a cure for every disease! But it's an individual cure based on the adjustment of a person's vibratory rate. In a world where opposites exist side by side — day and night, male and female, ease and dis-ease — there is always the potential for healing according to the spiritual laws of Nature. In this book, Paul Twitchell shows you how to discover your personal pathway to greater health and well-being, greater longevity, and a more youthful body.

Each day, we have a choice . . . to build a more healthy, youthful, aware future or allow the destruction of health and longevity by the inertia of daily living. Here are the keys to understanding your health, your personal body type, the role of disease in your spiritual growth, and the specific herbs and foods which balance inherited weaknesses. And most importantly, *Herbs: The Magic Healers* carries you past the confusion and conflicting opinions so prevalent in the health field to where you can know what's right for you!

Sri Harold Klemp, the current Living ECK Master, is releasing this new edition in 1986 — the Year of Spiritual Healing. *Herbs: The Magic Healers* can show you how to discover the only true healing in all the worlds of God . . . Spiritual Healing. To heal your body is a noble undertaking, for it is an active expression in your life of the ECK, the Living Word. A healthy body and mind enhance every moment of life and can help you reach God-Realization.

This book does more than open the door to the world of herbs. It takes you beyond herbology to an understanding of the very life processes that govern the use of herbs. Provocative insights into the many aspects of health, nutrition, and herbs make this book universal in its appeal. Its ageless wisdom holds the secret of the magic herbs that may revitalize you.

This special edition of *Herbs: The Magic Healers* has been reviewed and supplemented by A. Stuart Wheelwright, master herbalist, nutritionist, and biochemist. Wheelwright is renowned for his work in categorizing herbs according to their energy fields and researching the laws which govern the combining of herbs.

1

Herbs, the Ancient Way to Physical and Spiritual Well-Being

Spiritual healing in Eckankar, the Ancient Science of Soul Travel, is done by the hoary method of *Atma* (Soul), or out-of-the-body, movement. Healing is but one aspect of Eckankar. Its primary purpose is to give Soul an opportunity to travel the ancient, secret path to the realm of God where It becomes a Co-worker with the SUGMAD, the Supreme Deity.

For thousands of years, herbs have been used by the Adepts of the Ancient Order of the Vairagi, the Masters of Eckankar, to correct the spiritual and physical conditions of their students.

During the ancient times, these Adepts taught their chelas where to find the proper herbs and how to use them to soothe the anguish of body and heart. These herbs brought about "magical" changes in the individual who needed a few ingredients to bring him back to well-being again.

1

However, the ancient formulas of herbs, spices, and minerals are still available. That is why this book on herbs is being made available today, so that all who do not have any contact with the Living ECK Master or other ECK Masters can have the opportunity to find release from physical and mental health problems.

The Living ECK Master does not depend upon herbs to bring about the adjustment from illness to health; he works with the individual according to his level of spiritual unfoldment. If one has developed far enough up the spiritual ladder of God, it requires little effort to heal the psychic wounds or illness of the physical self.

Modern medicine was founded upon herbs, plants, flowers, minerals, and spices. We know that through the study of herbs new ingredients for the healing of man's mind and body are being found in the jungles of South America and other parts of the world. The Living ECK Master is gradually leading man to those places where herbs grow wild in order to help raise bodily health conditions. Every ECK Master follows the old axiom in Eckankar: "It is better to have a healthy body when trying to reach God-Realization than one filled with pain, anguish, and sickness." It is taught that one concentrates better upon God or any subjective experience in life with a healthy mind and body.

The Living ECK Master also teaches that what is good for one individual in herb healing may not be especially so for another; everyone cannot use the same herbs for the same results. Each person is different in his consciousness and in his body metabolism.

Therefore, we must accept the fact that whatever one person can use and benefit from may not be best for everyone. Generally speaking, one formula for an herb mixture produces a remedy for numerous people; but in the long run, there is no sure, single prescription for everyone. If a person needs a diagnosis or a prescription for a specific health problem, he should see his own physician, who can handle his case according to the laws of medicine.

Aristotle, the great Greek philosopher, left a book, *Golden Cabinet of Secrets,* which was composed of many formulas, recipes, and prescriptions regarding certain herbs and plants that he and his contemporaries had studied. He found many plants to be poisonous and narcotic in nature, so his works were kept secret. Certain highly influential politicians of his time would not have hesitated to use such herbs and plants for the degradation of many of the people, so Aristotle passed the information on only to the more trustworthy of his followers.

Aristotle discovered herbs that were astringents and had the property of contracting tissue. He also found antispasmodics, which helped prevent spasms and relieved muscular irritability. He found demulcents, which soothed the membranes of the nose and throat, helping coughs and colds.

The philosopher wrote voluminously about tonics, sedatives, aromatics, laxatives, and purgatives. Many famous people of history used the recipes which Aristotle put together, including Alexander the Great and Cleopatra.

The magic of herbs wove its spell over the people of the Middle Ages. The witches were the greatest advocates of herbal medicines and magic. Satan, the Prince of Darkness, was supposed to possess mysterious powers gained from a concoction he brewed during those Dark Ages. He has apparently retired from this area of influence and now works spells with the Kal (negative) power over the hearts and minds of the people in modern times.

The peoples of the Middle Ages believed there was magic in the herbal philters. Herbs and plants were the basis of the love potions and aphrodisiacs. These potions were used in every way—sometimes given as a liquid to drink and at other times poured over various parts of the body; for example, on the soles of the feet.

The ancient writings of Aristotle, Democritus, Paracelsus, Albertus Magnus, and others included many recipes for love powders and philters. During the time of Queen Elizabeth I, the roots of the eryngo, the sea holly, were used as a love tonic. During the Renaissance, love potions made from herbs became a thriving business.

Percy Shelley, the great English poet, used many herbal concoctions during his search for eternal youth in Italy. He often mixed his own herbs in order to develop the right recipe to make himself youthful. Lord Byron, his companion in Italy, helped in the search, but neither seemed to have found the secret recipe for physical immortality, as both died quite young. Shelley died by drowning, Byron of a fever.

In the past, wandering tribes were most knowledgeable in herbs, and they depended upon them for survival. The wisdom of plant lore was handed down through the ages from generation to generation. It

4

was especially true of the tribes in the Far East, mostly those in China where herbs still hold great value.

The ECK Masters have realized that it is not the knowledge of a large number of herbs that brings the greatest botanical benefit for people, but the thorough knowledge of a few of the better ones. Thorough knowledge includes how herbs should be prepared, blended, and mixed so that they are compatible with one another and augment one another to keep from reducing individual effectiveness.

One learns not to blend certain incompatible herbs. For example, yellow dock root, a blood tonic, would not be mixed with oak bark, because the tannic acid in the latter and iron in the former are incompatible with one another. Tannic acid united with iron forms tannate of iron which produces intestinal disorders and constipation.

An individual can survive quite well on a pound of food each day — even less if the food has been carefully selected. The principal abuse in eating is the consumption of excessive amounts of starch and glutinous foods — too much bread, cooked cereals, potatoes, macaroni, spaghetti, all beans (except string beans), peas, lentils, pies, cakes, pastry, blancmange, thick soups, gravies, chocolate milks and foods of similar nature.

If eaten in excess these mucous and acid-forming foods do not perfectly digest and they will ferment in the digestive tract, forming alcohol and acetic acid. They tend to clog the mucous membranes and produce catarrhs, colds, and bowel troubles.

One of the points which the ECK Masters tried to get across to the ECK chelas (students) during

5

ancient times was that calcium chloride is a great nutrient for the heart. Medical support for such an assertion was discovered several years ago by medical scientists in England. An herb containing calcium chloride, such as motherwort, may help avert heart problems. By some mysterious process, motherwort can draw calcium and chlorine out of the soil and convert it into a calcium chloride that is nontoxic and can be used by the heart to help it function better. Calcium is used by the muscles of the heart to help them relax so they can rebuild. It is said that the heart consumes enormous amounts of calcium chloride.

There are several herbal heart remedies, each seemingly designed for some specific condition of the heart. The family of lime plants which helps the heart so much seems to be able to take advantage of certain waste elements and convert them into nourishing foods.

Another herb used in the treatment of heart trouble is the hawthorn apple. Formerly regarded as sacred (traditionally it furnished Jesus' crown of thorns) it was chosen by Henry VII of England as part of his coat of arms. The hawthorn apple is called *Crataegus oxyacantha* from the Greek word meaning hard, sharp thorn.

The hawthorn, known as thorn apple tree, may tree, white thorn, or haws thorn tree, is a long-lived tree growing to a height of about thirty feet. It produces a small fruit about a half inch in diameter. These are borne in great numbers and are deep red to purplish black. The fruit is used as a diuretic, astringent, nervine, and tonic for sore throats. The American Indians used the fruit to strengthen weak hearts, as a survival food, and to make pemmican. Dried meat, dried haws, and fat were pounded together, stored, and used when traveling great distances.

Common sense tells us that nature supplies most of our foods from the vegetable and herb kingdom and that it supplies the remedies for most illnesses. Every animal has an inborn instinct and, when sick, will seek out certain grasses, weeds, or plants to eat. We owe a great deal to the American Indians and natives of other countries, who, through the centuries, learned how to cure their ailments with herbs. Science now confirms through chemical analysis the fact that all the chemical elements of which our body is composed are also found in the roots, barks, leaves, flowers, and fruits of herbs.

We have also learned that each family of plants and herbs has its own peculiar ability for extracting from the earth a specific group of mineral elements. The lime plants, which are the legumes, peas, beans, clovers, etc., supply calcium, potassium, phosphorus, and similar minerals which are the materials to build bones, ligaments, and teeth. The lily family stores organic sulfur, as do legumes, peas, beans, etc. These are important to the diet, supplying the sulfur-bearing amino acids. These are called essential amino acids because they cannot be manufactured in the human body, but must be supplied in the food eaten. They make up hormones, enzymes, liver cells, spleen cells, and play an essential part in sight and taste. The sulfur-bearing amino acids also play an important function in detoxification of the tissues.

The iron plants, rubus, yellow, or curled, dock, raisins, almonds, spinach, etc., all supply an

7

abundance of the essential element iron used by the body to build red blood cells (hemoglobin). This is necessary to provide an adequate supply of oxygen to all the organs and tissues. Yellow dock root is a very good source of iron, and some women take a teaspoon or two during menstruation to resupply the iron lost. This is an excellent supplier of iron that does not cause constipation. Chlorophyll and yellow dock supply all the factors needed by the body to build hemoglobin which is similar to chlorophyll but contains a molecule of iron, where chlorophyll contains magnesium.

The phosphorous plants — grains and seeds — contain phosphorus in the form of lecithin, a phospholipid which makes a very assimilable, usable phosphorous substance essential for nerve and brain function. Also, the body must maintain a ratio of four units of phosphorus for each ten units of calcium and 0.1 unit of manganese.

Within the plant kingdom we find not only food materials, but tonics, laxatives, astringents, stimulants, sedatives, and every element needed to balance the body chemistry, to overcome body ills and bring about health.

The following list gives many herbs according to their need and properties for the body. This is not a complete list because space does not allow it.

The amulet herbs. These are used by many people who believe in their occult value to bring "good luck." Some of these herbs have medicinal properties, but they are used primarily because of their alleged benefit to the seeker of good fortune. Often the herbs are sewn into a bag and carried around the

8

neck. Some people merely place a bag of these herbs in their purse or carry them in a pocket somewhere on their person.

These herbs are as follows: Adam and Eve root, alkanet root, betel nut, buckeye, cumin seed, devil's shoestrings, five-finger grass, grains of paradise, high John the Conqueror, holy herb, sandalwood, lesser periwinkle, life everlasting, lovage root, queen's root, sacred bark, sumbul root, tonka bean, and wahoo bark.

The anthelmintic herbs. It is said these herbs rid the body of tapeworms and other types of parasitic worms in the stomach and intestines. This type of complaint is common among those, who in their search for independence, become unkempt and neglectful of body sanitation. It is also common among young people, especially those who surf and go barefooted much of the time in warm climates such as Florida, California and the Southwest, and the southern United States.

Parasitic worms have reached a pandemic proportion. These are usually referred to as nematodes. It has been reported that sixty million people have nematode infections due to exposure to pets. Forty-five million people have pork trichinosis, and in some areas of the United States, such as Arizona, Montana, and South Dakota where tests have been run, up to eighty-two percent of the people have some kind of nematode infection.

There are estimated to be 500,000 species of nematodes, although most are not parasites. They may vary from being so small that it takes a microscope to see them, to tapeworms that may be over twenty feet long. They may come from uncooked foods, going barefoot (animal droppings), handshakes, toilets, doorknobs, fruit (skin contaminated by handlers), raw fish (sashimi), handling or eating raw or undercooked meat or improperly cooked pork which has three major tape nematodes. Trichinosis, which affects the spine, muscles, and nerves, is extremely painful, contributing to arthritis (often misdiagnosed). Nematodes that live in the large intestine, seven inches long and a quarter inch across, may proliferate to the thousands. Porcine tapeworms that are paper thin and three-fourths of an inch wide may grow up to sixty feet long.

Dog heartworms are possible in those who have dogs, especially if the dogs are allowed to run free. The worms get into the heart and perforate the heart muscles causing heart failure. They are wire-thin, about 1 1/2 inches long, and may number in the tens of thousands.

Brain nematodes may be the cause of insanity, irrationality, debility, blindness, deafness, deformity problems, or rheumatoid arthritis. Nematodes can cause migratory aches and pains, skin rashes, muscle cramps, constipation, dysentery, lung problems, allergies, liver complaints, impotency, gastritis, ulcerations, body aches, sciatica, crippled and deformed joints, bloating, bulging abdomen, overweight, underweight, lethargy, fatigue, short temper, chronic indigestion, bumps, growths, etc.

In China, everyone cooks everything they eat. Doctors say that it is necessary as all the plants harvested for food or medicine have been fertilized with night soil (human dung), and the soil is infested with nematodes which would infect the people who eat the plants.

Eating only cooked food damages the liver and spleen and congests the lymphatic system. This is why ginseng helps them so much. Ginseng is the best lymph decongester of all herbs. On the other hand we in the West have very little lymphatic congestion, and so ginseng is not as effective an herb for us. Because we live and eat differently, we have different needs.

Very few United States doctors have anything to do with nematodes or recognize the symptoms, and their cure is often worse than the infection.

We shake hands with someone who perhaps didn't wash after toileting or handling raw meat, animal dung, etc., then we sooner or later transfer the infection by rubbing our eyes. This picks up the egg and carries it into the nasal passage where it hatches and starts to grow. Or, perhaps a cat or dog licks our hand, and then we rub our eye. Or someone coughs near us and the droplets carry a viable nematode to our eye. Or dust blows into our eye; this dust could have come from infested animal dung.

There is some belief that some of these parasites may be transmitted venereally. Adult nematodes may be so small that 600 of them could live on a period ("."); the egg could be hundreds of times smaller.

Water may also carry parasites. Liver flukes from contaminated water are very prevalent in the South and even up into Montana. Spraying Chlorox over the contaminated water and continuing to its source, may easily wipe it out. It is said that drinking six drops of Chlorox in a glass of water, once a day for four or five days will clean up this pest. This seems to work for most animals that are involved with this pesky nematode.

Through the Asian, south Asian, and South American countries, and Mexico, there are two rather drastic herbs used to expel nematodes — halpa de jalpa and zopilopatle. These are drastic herbs and must be used with care. Only a very small amount will do the job.

Parasitic worms constitute a problem in India where it is often customary to go without shoes, especially among the religious there. Most so-called holy men and religious seekers in India are bothered by worms because of a lack of body sanitation.

While on this point, it is well to inform those who always believe what is being taught in the Orient as truth in religious and spiritual matters, of the conditions in ashrams and monasteries. These ingenuous people would be startled to know that most of these places are filled with disease and sex perversions. Few ashrams in the Orient are kept up to the standards of Western sanitation. As a result, the occupants live in filth and disease. Many of the young priests are taught to be celibates, but nothing is said about self-abuse.

The herbs in the anthelmintic category that are available to us are many, probably well over a hundred. A few of these are wormseed, pomegranate, pumpkin seed, walnut hulls, kamala, quassia chips, betel nut, white oak bark, butternut, hops, garlic, sage, and peach leaves. Lemon leaves are good when used alone.

Parents may "deworm" children by using garlic as follows: One teaspoon garlic powder (from the grocery store); with one tablespoon molasses. Use one-third of this mixture every three days, three times. This will get rid of pinworms. If children are especially restless and grind their teeth at night while sleeping, it may be pinworms.

Most parasites are difficult to deal with. Getting rid of the adults is the easiest part of the job. They go through three stages: eggs, extremely small; larvae, which can burrow through tissue and move through the body; and adults, which generally localize (stay in one place), often attaching to the walls of the colon. Destroying these parasites is far more complicated than destroying other infections since only the adult worms are affected by most anthelmintic herbs. It takes time for the larvae to mature and become adults, and still more time for the eggs to become adults. Some may take thirty-two days to go through a cycle. The adults seem to give off a controlling chemical that retards the development of competitors. So, when the adults are flushed out of the colon, this control is lost and others may begin to develop. So, should you start a program, be sure to complete it.

Follow it for ten days, then stop for five days. This will allow your body to correct and adjust. Then, on for ten days and off for five days. Do this cycle at least four to six times. This will get the adults, larvae, and eggs. Anything less will allow the parasites to reinfest.

So, remember the cycle: 10−5−10−5−10−5−10−5.

The aromatic or carminative herbs. These are generally pleasant and pungent to the taste. They are often used to make other drugs more palatable and to prevent griping in cathartics. Their use is to rid the body of stomach and intestinal gases.

These herbs are as follows: angelica root, anise root, caraway, cardamom seed, catnip, celery seed, coriander seed, cumin seed, elecampane root, parsley root, peppermint, spearmint, sweet clover, wild ginger, raisins, and fennel seed.

Mixed with a meal these often prevent gases from arising in the stomach and intestines. The ECK Masters have long used these as an aid to good digestion and have recommended them to the chelas of the true spiritual works. They help to keep the body in good health and are part of the botanicals used in our daily lives.

Some people say that if they eat five or six raisins, twenty minutes before a meal, their indigestion clears up and they are never bothered with gas or heartburn.

In the East and Near East, a small bowl is often passed around, and each person in turn takes a pinch of fennel seeds or anise seeds (five to eight) and chews them thoroughly. In Mexico, it is the common custom to use a salsa made of anise, garlic, hot pepper, and tomato sauce. Perhaps a tablespoon of this is consumed at the very beginning of a meal to stimulate the flow of gastric juices, and generally it is used on corn tortillas during the meal.

The astringent herbs. These are herbs used for botanical formulas to contract the tissues of the body when the physician deems it necessary.

They are as follows: alumroot, bilberry, black alder bark, blackberry bark, wild cherry, black willow bark, butternut bark, hawthorn, kola nuts, pearl-

14

flowered life everlasting, golden maidenhair, mountain ash fruit, white pond lily root, white oak root, and sweet fern leaves.

The herbs used in dyes and coloring. These herbs were first used by the primitive Indian tribes in North America for dyeing clothes and coloring headdresses. Later they were put to use in the cosmetic industry for toilet preparations, hair tonics, and dyes in textile mills and garment factories where women's and men's clothes are assembled for retail sales.

These herbs and the colors they produce are as follows: alkanet — red; bloodroot — red; blue malva — blue; henna leaves — yellow; goldenseal — yellow; madder — red; sage — green; saffron — yellow; sumac leaves — yellow; sumac root — black; red saunders — red; and walnut leaves — brown.

You can see that it was relatively easy for the primitive tribesman to find colors in the herbs of the fields and forest whenever he wanted to dye any of his clothing or implements such as arrows, weapons, or feathers.

The diuretic herbs. These are used in medicines to flush the kidneys and promote the secretion of urine. Generally, they are used when the kidneys are not active enough.

These herbs are as follows: birch sap, burdock seeds, corn silk, couch grass, American dwarf elder bark, horseradish root, juniper berries, kava kava, parsley root, scarlet pimpernel, pipsissewa, seven barks, trailing arbutus, and watermelon seed.

The problem here is that most people have a tendency to use diuretics to an excess, thus overstimulating the kidneys.

15

The expectorants. These herbs tend to modify the quality and quantity of the mucus secretions and favor its expulsion in case of colds, coughs, and irritations of the throat.

The expectorant herbs are as follows: balm of Gilead fir, butterfly weed, horehound, pearl-flowered life everlasting, greater nettle leaves, seneca root, Solomon's seal, wahoo bark, wild cherry bark, and white pine bark.

These are the chief ingredients used in medicines for colds and coughs. They were first used by the medicine man in the primitive tribes, especially the American Indians. They were found in the medicine chests of the early settlers in this country.

The fragrant herbs. The fragrant botanicals are used in sachet perfumes, incense mixtures, and in the manufacture of certain flavors. The ancient Persians and Greeks were heavy users of these herbs, as were the Chinese.

They are as follows: cassia bark, cloves, deer's tongue leaves (wild vanilla), myrrh gum, lavender flowers, orris root, pennyroyal, peppermint, sandalwood, sweet woodruff, rose petals, tansy, tonka bean, wild ginger, and wintergreen.

The laxative herbs. These are the herbs which stimulate the secretions of the intestines and excite the movement of the bowels. They are the basis for the patent medicines found so commonly on drugstore shelves today, known simply as laxatives.

The laxative herbs are as follows: butternut, cascara sagrada, dandelion root, mountain flax seed, goldenseal, licorice root, rhubarb root, senna pod, snakehead, and St. John's bread.

Nervine herbs have a soothing effect on the nerves, and were used in the past as the basis of many patent medicines.

These herbs are as follows: scullcap, vervain, celery seed, valerian, hop flower, kola nuts, lady's slipper, mistletoe, mugwort, musk root, rosemary, sweet basil, and wild lettuce.

The purgative herbs. These are similar to the laxatives, except they are far stronger and induce a much heavier action on the bowels. They are also found to form a base for patent medicines.

These herbs are as follows: black root, boneset, buckthorn bark, may apple root, and senna leaves.

The tonic herbs. They are divided into two parts: Those called simply tonics and used primarily by women for their particular needs. Secondly, those called stomachics which promote nutrition and tone up the stomach for loss of appetite.

The tonic herbs are as follows: alder, angelica, bearberry, bethroot, blue cohosh, elecampane root, life root, lovage, saw palmetto berries, queen's delight, rosemary, shepherd's purse, squaw vine, and tansy.

The stomachic herbs are as follows: angelica root, blackberry root, gentian, chicory root, chocolate root, calumba, dandelion root, elecampane, ginseng root, goldenseal, Jamaica ginger, juniper berries, mugwort root, quassia, Solomon's seal, basil, thyme, sage, and wild strawberry.

The herbs so named are some of those which make up the botanicals. These are the plants, flowers, and herbs that are used in medical prescriptions and patent medicines. But we must remember that much of the real value of herbs has been lost through the centuries from ancient times because many have become domesticated, garden types.

Agriculture began in the ancient East in the region of Anatolia, Syria, and Mesopotamia. In the Western world it began in Mexico. In both of these regions it started near the end of the last ice age, about 10,000 years ago. In both regions it began with the cultivation of plants and extended later to the herding of animals.

The development of man from the Neolithic era to the present day could be viewed through the history of plants. Plants certainly have had an influence upon man. Because of lost nutrients in plants, flowers, and herbs today, we are resorting to artificial means to assist the body in its struggle in this earth world. During the latter years and into the modern age, the chemical laboratory has brought about changes in modern man.

Wild grain in ancient times gave a high-yielding bread wheat that contained more of the body-building ingredients than the wheat of today. During the twenties and thirties, wheat production was threatened with a smut plague that nearly wiped out our major grain crop. The scientists found smut resistant varieties. These varieties had a toxic membrane around the kernel that would not let the smut grow. They bred this membrane onto nearly all our grain. This wheat causes more allergic reactions, and its nutritional value is severely altered. It is possible to remove this membrane electronically, but it would cost more. So, we consume this toxic substance in our food. Some varieties such as Blue Stem Bart wheat from Idaho have not been inbred and do not have this toxic membrane.

The interbreeding of races also brought about changes in the cultivation of grain and other products. It meant changes in locations as tribes moved to other places. About five thousand years ago as the farmers spread into new lands, met the hunters, and produced new families of hunters, farmers, and herders, the movements into Europe and Egypt called for adaptations of crops, stock, and people. We find that some grains, herbs, and plants grow better in certain farming areas. For example, rye grows better in the highlands rather than in ground at a low level. Rice in lowlands has a richer quality than in the highlands.

The new breed of agriculturists brought with them new ideas and methods which in turn affected the nutrient content in the field and farm products. Grains, plants, herbs, and flowers, the botanicals which were the ancestors of the ingredients used in modern medicines, began to lose their natural properties. Today, they do not possess the same powerful ingredients.

The pedigree of herbs was lost in the crossbreeding and transplanting from different areas. These plants have been so robbed of their natural properties that little has been left in the ingredients being used today. We find few herbs growing wild in countries maintaining a high civilization.

Natural herbs are still found in an abundance in parts of South America. Some scientists believe that

19

the Amazon valley, covering parts of Peru, Colombia, Ecuador, Bolivia, and Brazil, is one of the few spots on this planet that has not experienced an Ice Age. Most of the rest of the world has been covered with ice many times. The ice builds up on the land to a depth of over a mile, slipping-sliding, wearing down mountains, cutting canyons, and reconditioning the land.

When the ice melts off, there is little if any vegetation. So, Amazonia has been a reseeding source. In all the world, outside of Amazonia, there are some 50,000 species of plants. About ten percent of them have some herbal value, and about 2,400 of these have been used by American herbalists and recorded in their literature. In Amazonia, there are thought to be nearly 300,000 species, and if ten percent of them have herbal qualities, that would be a potential of forty to fifty thousand herbs.

Actually, seventy-five percent of all foods eaten in the United States and Europe have come from South America in the past hundred or so years. Examples are corn, peppers, melons, bananas, tapioca, tomatoes, potatoes, beans, squash, etc. All have found their way into our diet. We would be hard-pressed if we had to live without them. The future of modern nutrition will draw upon the abundance found in that strange and beautifully productive land. There are thousands of plants that could be used by the world to bring health and abundance to mankind.

Most of the natural herbs grow in the South American jungles and in Africa. A few grow in the highlands of China, and they can be picked wild on the slopes of the Himalayan foothills in northern India and in Tibet. There are herb hunters just as there are orchid seekers, both braving the jungles for their precious botanical quarry.

Scientists have given little thought to this evolution of plants, the average man even less. But it is important for us to realize that reincarnation and karmic patterns of life are involved here, similar to that of the Soul which inhabits the human body. A plant has a consciousness, even though it only expresses itself simply, whereas man expresses himself in more complex ways.

We find that plants respond to the seasons, as does man. Man is subject to the seasonal availability of plants, or he must provide some method by which they can be dried, preserved, or stored safely in order to be consumed during an off-season period.

Today we eat too many artificial products developed in the laboratories, too many processed foods with preservatives detrimental to our health. In addition we are not free from the poisonous effects of the sprays used to rid crops of insects.

We have those who say that if we think right and hold good thoughts, nothing can harm us, and we will have good health. This is not always true because we are dealing with bacteria, viruses, fungi, and parasites which have a destroying power if our bodies are not healthy enough to counteract the attack upon bodily tissue.

Throughout the ages, man has been far more interested in herbs possessing magic ingredients which might give him a great love attraction or bring him good fortune. He has seldom connected the herb with his health. Only a few informed people — the

21

medicine man, witch, alchemist, apothecary, monk, and philosopher—have had the knowledge to make use of the herbs and plants, and they commonly put some religious restrictions upon their use, rather than using them for beneficial health reasons.

There were many who used mixtures of herbs to be carried on their person. At first these were carried in a small bag around the neck. Later, herbs were put into a jeweled receptacle which took the form of a heart and was called an amulet of love. Some of these amulet herbs have already been listed.

Sandalwood mixed with rose water is still used in some parts of India during the middle of April by women who sprinkle the mixture on everyone they meet. This symbolizes the washing away of the impurities of the old year and the starting of the new year without sin.

We find that herbs are given space in *The Shariyat-Ki-Sugmad,* the holy writings of Eckankar. Herbs are also mentioned several times in the various sacred religious writings of the world.

Prominent is the balm of Gilead, from the small tree, the balsam of Gilead, native to the Middle Eastern countries. This herb is found in the mountains of Gilead east of the Holy Land. It yields the celebrated balm, a resinous substance obtained by making incisions in the tree. When first tapped, the substance is white, but once exposed to air, it turns a golden color and looks much like honey.

In ancient times there was a legend of magical significance attached to the balm of Gilead. It was thought to be so potent that if a person coated his hands with it, he could hold them over fire without harm.

So many of the negative emotions can be handled by anyone in good health. Many people do not understand that health is the first factor on the road to God-Realization. If one is in good health, one is better able to do spiritual exercises than if one suffers from pain and anguish.

Most of the curatives on the drug counters today are not directly from the herbs of the fields, mountains, and woods, but from the test tube. The trouble here is that few of these artificial nostrums have the full curative powers for the diseases which attack modern man today.

During the first quarter of this century there was an organized move away from the use of herbs and natural methods in medicine. Research based on the use and development of drugs composed of chemicals derived from the petroleum industry became dominant. The emphasis on chemicals stopped development of most herbal products. Nearly all herbs were eventually dropped from the United States pharmacies, and petroleum-derived drugs were substituted. The Federal Drug Administration (FDA) furthered this process by requiring strict labeling of the contents of products. The actual potencies of natural products could not be uniformly maintained batch after batch, as nutrients in a vegetable product may vary according to when and where it is grown and harvested. So, vitamin companies were forced to use mostly synthetic sources.

In the herb kingdom we find the most remarkable combinations of elements which suit every requirement of the human system. Just why the researchers for the chemical laboratories do not turn more fully to herbs, plants, flowers, and similar things is puzzling. Not only do herbs supply food materials, but tonics, laxatives, astringents, stimulants, sedatives, diuretics, stone dissolvers, and every element needed to balance the body chemistry and overcome disease.

A lifetime is required to learn the names, nature, and habits of the hundreds of thousands of plants that compose the herb kingdom. It would take several thousand years to learn the medicinal or the therapeutic nature of a comparatively small number of them. But the future holds promise that within the next fifty years we shall double or triple the national knowledge of herbs. Thus we shall help resolve the problems of disease and considerably lengthen the span of life on earth.

2

The Restoration of Spiritual Health through Herbs

The restoration of spiritual health through herbs should be a goal of every individual in his life.

By speaking of the spiritual health of man, I do not talk about body tissue or the things that make up only the physical well-being of the individual. I speak of the mental and the emotional, which are the elements that make up the psychic and Soul faculties of man. Once we have established good health in these areas, the physical aspect of man is bound to improve and bloom in exceedingly wondrous ways.

It is in these inner planes of man that many are able to find themselves advancing rapidly on the path to spiritual unfoldment and, eventually, God-Realization. Man first becomes aware of himself, which is Self-Realization, then gains knowledge of Soul, and later God-Realization, which is the knowledge of God. The use of the proper foods and herbs will assist in the spiritual unfoldment of every individual.

In the East, herbal treatment is known to have been used long before the era of Hippocrates. The *Pen-Ts'ao Kang Mu,* the great herbal book of China, is a compilation of herbal knowledge that was in use about three thousand years before the beginning of Christianity. Among the oldest books on medical remedies, it went into much detail about the use of herbal medicines.

Another manuscript, older than the *Pen-Ts'ao Kang Mu,* was the *Ebers Papyrus,* dating from 1500 B.C., which lists over eight hundred herbal remedies, including castor oil. Parts of *The Shariyat-Ki-Sugmad,* the original sacred writings of Eckankar, include discussions of many herbs, plants, and flowers. Pliny states in his *Natural History* that he believed there was an herbal remedy for every physical disorder.

The herbalists have never claimed that their herbs could cure in the same sense that antibiotics or allopathics do, by killing germs or destroying toxic poisons in the body. All an herb, or its distilled essence, can do is assist the body by stimulating its resistance to attacks upon its tissues.

The herbs work in mysterious ways. There are herbs that stimulate and others that sedate. Some do both — first stimulating, later sedating. When an organ or tissue is stimulated, it will throw off the toxic wastes that build up through metabolism. When relaxed, nature takes over and rebuilds. Everything that is living or has lived, has a life energy force within its molecular makeup. There are herbs that contain specific energy forces of the same nature as the energy forces found in tissues or organs. In other words, an herb that has a certain energy level will affect the nerves of the body which also have that same energy level.

Our knowledge of DNA (deoxyribonucleic acid) explains a lot about herbs and how and why they function. DNA is made up of two microscopic strands which form a loose spiral, the double helix. Stretched out, these strands would be a yard long, but in Nature they generally form a spiral within a spiral within a spiral, etc. They are so very compact that forty-six of them will fit into the nucleus of a human cell. When stretched out, this spiral would appear like a railroad track; two parallel tracks held together and apart by 40,000 railroad ties. Each of these ties is made up of nucleotides which carry data. The human cell, when it is first fertilized, contains enough information to reproduce an entire human body.

A plant that for instance is effective in healing the heart, has within its cellular structure the DNA data to reestablish the genetic structure of the heart and re-educate the heart to its proper function.

For each of the forty-four major body organs there are herbs which have the necessary data to renew man's body season by season. Herbs contain not just vitamins or minerals but are the architects of the organs and contain the blueprints needed to restore the lost information that the body requires to reconstruct the damage brought on by accidents, poor diet, poor inheritance, or old age.

When an organ is under stress, diseased. or damaged, the DNA breaks down into smaller groups of genes that tend to congest in various places — which interferes with the body's ability to rebuild. The

27

proper herbs can restore or reeducate these sick cells and organs so that they function properly.

When you combine herbs it is essential that you know which herb does what to the DNA. It may take six to twenty herbs to supply the necessary data to restructure an organ.

We are just on the threshold of knowledge when it comes to herbology. It is the oldest science and also the newest.

Interwoven with the legends and myths of time and history is the truth about herbs. For example, we have the account of the mysterious manna which fell from heaven for the wandering Israelites as they fled from the Egyptians. In truth, this was an herbal agent which was the product of the tamarisk, a tree that secretes a juice through its bark. It is valued as a healing herb, but because of its agreeable taste it was considered food from heaven by the wandering tribe of Israel. Another "manna" which they found and ate was the coriander seed.

Herbs like spikenard, frankincense, and myrrh were generally used in ancient times as incense and perfume with the special property of centering the mind on devotion and producing an elevated mental state. Such a heightened state of consciousness in turn affects the psychic senses and increases the phenomena of psychic awareness.

Myrrh is that herb given to arouse the spiritual senses in man. It is probably valued above all other herbs as an incense ingredient. It was, in ancient times, mixed with benzoin. The ECK Masters have used it at times to help a chela become spiritually aroused so that he can gain some experience of survival through Soul Travel. This is not a general practice, however, for the ECK Masters of the Ancient Order of the Vairagis want the chela to learn Soul Travel by his own conscious volition, and not by having to lean upon something like myrrh or other props to get out of his physical senses into the spiritual worlds.

Hyssop is another herb which was, and still is, used in the religious worlds. It was mainly used in the early days as a symbol of purification. Later it was discovered to be valuable as a healing agent for the wounds of warriors injured in battle or in accidents.

The wound was dressed with hyssop leaves as a protection against infection and to promote healing. This was done in the beginning with a crude effectiveness, but then the physicians and nurses became more proficient. This herb was the object of much superstition until modern medical researchers found that the mold which grows on the hyssop leaves produced a kind of natural penicillin.

Today some 350,000 known herbs and plants have been examined and classified and approximately 4,000 new species are added to the list yearly. Yet man still does not understand the potential of these herbs and plants for maintaining the health of the individual.

One herb, which has never become too popular with the general public, except for the Italians, is common garlic. For over five thousand years it has been used to cure many ailments. As far back as

3000 B.C., the Babylonians knew and used garlic as a curative aid. The physicians and priests in ancient Egypt fed garlic to the thousands of slaves that worked on the Cheops pyramid in order to keep up their strength. The Phoenicians and Vikings carried large amounts of garlic with them on their sea voyages.

Garlic is so important that during the First World War, the British government made a desperate call to the public for all the garlic they could provide. As a result thousands of tons were bought for the purpose of treating wounds of the troops returning from France and the front lines. It helped to prevent infection and healed wounds more rapidly.

It is said that among the thousands of wounded men treated with garlic not one case of infection was found. Others have stated that it helps in the treatment of tuberculosis. However accurate these reports may be, garlic is known to lower blood pressure, clear the skin of pimples, abscesses, boils, carbuncles, and ulcers.

Herbs are special in the sense that the SUGMAD (God) made them for a purpose, and that purpose must have been for the healing of the embodiment of man and to separate Soul and body—to give Soul Its opportunity to travel in the other worlds, provided It could do this in no other way.

One must heal himself before attending to anything else. He must undertake a rigid regimen in which all foods consumed are the ECK (positive) foods. Too much emphasis is placed upon the Kal (negative) foods, and they have become the bane of civilization.

Government reports link cancer and heart disease with cigarettes and tobacco smoking, but little or no mention is ever made of the Kal foods and drinks.

The Kal foods and drinks include tea, coffee, tobacco, refined sugar, alcoholic beverages, soft drinks, and chocolate. Recreational drugs are also Kal substances. Each of these has a damaging effect on the total body energy. Every person has a certain energy level. Two tablespoons of a soft drink may reduce this energy level by half for three to six hours. On the other hand, a selection of raw, leafy vegetables (not head lettuce, tomatoes, or the skins of cucumbers), fish (shrimp, scallops, conch), and some seeds or sprouts, will quickly double that energy level.

There are some foods that are predominately Kal. A few of them have already been mentioned. The following is a more complete list of foods that can deplete the body's energy.

tea (non-herbal)
coffee
tobacco
alcoholic beverages
soft drinks
iceberg lettuce
tomatoes
cucumber skins
homogenized milk
hydrogenated fats
white flour products

processed, preserved, or
    canned foods
high sugar foods
artificially-colored foods
food grown on
    chemically-treated or
    depleted soil
irradiated foods
synthetic vitamins
high carbohydrate foods

31

Some foods support and enhance a person's energy level. For example:

sprouts — alfalfa, clove, radish, mung, etc. (not soy)

fresh vegetables — green, leafy, peppers, peas

fish — conch, shrimp (fresh), octopus, scallops, red snapper and other fish from the cold, deep oceans

seeds — sunflower, squash, sesame, flax, chia, pumpkin

herbs — parsley, purslane, shepherd's purse, young rye and wheat grass

beverage herb teas for pleasure — spearmint, desert herb, chamomile, red clover, goldenrod, raspberry leaf, oat straw, horsetails

juices (dilute all fruit and vegetable juice with at least one-third water)

chicken occasionally

Remember, the foods you can grow yourself are your best food. Those grown locally are better than those grown in a distant place. Fresh is better than stored. Raw is usually better than cooked. Fresh is better than frozen. Frozen is better than canned. Anything that is done to a food from the time it is mature in the garden will destroy some of the value of the food — anything — storing, cooking, freezing, drying, etc.

It is surprising how little food is necessary to run the body. If you were to dehydrate and weigh all the food going into the body, and dehydrate and weigh the waste products given off by the body, you would find only a few ounces of difference in weight.

If one will stay on a rice diet of any sort, especially brown rice, for ten days or more, his health will improve. Then he can gradually go back to a balanced diet consisting of ECK and Kal foods. It is necessary to eliminate the impurities in the physical body first, then begin the balanced diet. It will help the physical system and give the mental faculties greater alertness.

Generally, after the fifth day of any ECK diet plan, one finds himself in a difficult state of health. His head aches; he may have diarrhea or may be very nauseated. All these are bodily protests against the purification plan. It is Kal's own way of trying to keep the body from throwing off the toxic poisons. The pain and aches result from the fact that the body does not want to turn loose any of its problems.

Once we revert to a diet that consists of hardly anything other than herbs, we find illness becoming a doorway to health, tragedy turning to comedy and disaster heralding blessings.

Avoid eating a meal in a restaurant unless you are able to select from the à la carte menu, where you are more likely to choose the type of herbs, fruits, and plants closer to your natural diet.

For centuries eating and drinking among the ECK chelas has been steeped in the ceremony of a traditional sacramental rite.

For the ECK chela, the kitchen and dining room have always been a sacred part of the home. Within those rooms is experienced one form of the basic and continuing mystery of life. Therein, the sacrifice of the plant and animal kingdom for the perpetuation of human life and thought is reenacted daily. All of

ECK, as far as its worldly continuation goes, is based upon the establishment of health and happiness, here and now. Of course, ECK deals with the hereafter, but it does not try to avoid what man has to do with his own responsibilities on earth today.

Without nourishment for the body, no life is possible. To eat in some form — whether it is like those particular ECK Masters of the Ancient Order of the Vairagis, the God-eaters, who partake of the ECK life force, or the man on the material level with two full meals a day — is to create new life for tomorrow through the sacrifice of the lower realms, including the herbal kingdom. Long ago it was learned that the body structure changes by eating, that the nature of man can be changed by what he eats and drinks. Therefore, eating and drinking are considered the most important rituals in the art of life, for they are involved in the creation of health and happiness.

Health and happiness means to be rid of fatigue and disease. To have a good appetite, good memory, good humor, and precision in thought and action. To be free from anxiety and fear. To have a great capacity for survival over illness and anxieties. To have joy, long life, and great spiritual adventures.

One does not need a great deal of sleep, but when he does, it should be sound, relaxed, and restful. Very few men can have great spiritual experiences with a diseased body and mind. It has happened, I grant you, but it is rarely the case, for most of us need sound health in order to have some sort of opportunity to do Soul Traveling or out-of-the-body movement.

For the building and maintaining of health, one's

food intake must contain minerals in a balanced supply.

First, there is *calcium,* which is essential for good bone structure, strong teeth, calm nerves, and good muscle tone. The body needs about one gram of calcium daily. The best natural sources of calcium are fresh fruits, vegetables, particularly green leafy vegetables, whole grains, milk, cheese, nuts, dark and blackstrap molasses, soybeans, soybean flour, and bone meal. Other sources include horsetails, toadflax, cleavers, parsley, meadowsweet, coltsfoot, pimpernel, plantain, silverweed, shepherd's purse, mistletoe, chamomile, dandelion, nettle leaves, and watercress.

Second, we need *chlorine,* which is a constituent of the acid in the gastric juice of the stomach. It aids in the purification and cleansing of the bodily system.

Chlorine stimulates the liver to act as a filter for waste products. It also is used in the production of hydrochloric acid in the stomach for digestion.

A deficiency of chlorine could cause the loss of hair and result in improper digestive power. It is found in kelp, dulse, leafy green vegetables, barley, ripe olives, and salt.

Third, we have *phosphorus,* which is equally good for the teeth and bone structure, as well as for brain tissue and the nervous system. Phosphorus is found in the structure of the nucleus of every body cell. It also assists in the maintenance of the acid-alkaline balance of the human body. Both calcium and phosphorus are necessary in the diet, for the former assists in the assimilation of phosphorus. Most of our foods do have phosphorus in large quantities, such as whole grains, dairy products, eggs, meat, beans, peas, nuts, and most fruits and vegetables. Other sources include calamus, caraway seeds, chickweed, meadowsweet, marigold flowers, licorice root, and dandelion.

Fourth, we find that *iron* is essential for building the red blood cells. These red blood cells have the responsibility of bringing oxygen to the cells of the body and taking away carbon dioxide. A deficiency of iron creates a lack of red blood cells and this brings about anemia and low blood pressure. It is the magnetic element which attracts oxygen.

Nearly all the foods which we eat have iron and oxygen. Wheat and most cereals contain iron in the form of iron phosphate, as do vegetables, such as beets, tomatoes, spinach, lettuce, cabbage, celery, carrots, turnips, squash, parsley, mustard greens, dandelion leaves, etc. But the principal source is in fruits. Other sources include yellow dock, nettle leaves, silverweed, rest harrow, burdock, toadflax, salep, mullein leaves, meadowsweet, devil's bit scabious, dandelion, sorrel, parsley, and dulse.

It might appear that some of this information is not connected with herbs, but it must be pointed out that all vegetables are herbs, whether they are called foods or medicines. We also must remember that minerals are the products of herbs and, therefore, must be considered in the study. It is also to be said that one ounce of prevention is worth a pound of cure, and whenever the chela can assimilate and keep

36

the fundamentals of herbal studies in mind, he will be more successful in attaining results.

Fifth is *iodine*. A tiny amount of this mineral is needed in the body to maintain the metabolic balance. This tiny bit of iodine is so important that it is better to take an oversupply than chance being undersupplied. The lack of iodine causes many deficiency symptoms such as goiter, unbalanced fat deposits, and even the appearance of stupidity. It is said that a tiny amount of this mineral can make the difference between a genius and an imbecile.

The thyroid gland located at the base of the throat regulates the body metabolism and requires small amounts of iodine daily to function properly. Iodine is found in seafoods, animal and vegetable products, cod liver oil, kelp, dulse, and raw sea salt. Other herbs include Irish moss, Iceland moss, and sarsparilla. All these plants are also a source of chlorine.

Most cod liver oil is highly refined, and if there is any iodine left in it, it would be a very small amount. However, if you can obtain freeze-dried fish liver, it is an excellent source.

The sixth mineral is *copper,* necessary for the proper utilization of iron in the body and the prevention of anemia. The best sources of copper are seafoods, liver, molasses, green leafy vegetables, soy products, egg yolk, whole grains, and fruits, particularly dried fruits. Apricots are especially rich in copper and iron. Raw potatoes and potato juice supply an excellent source of easily assimilated, organic copper. Other sources include alfalfa, cabbage, lettuce, spinach, kale.

The seventh mineral is *sodium,* which keeps the body in acid-alkaline balance and is necessary to keep calcium in solution for body needs. Salt, which is sodium chloride, is the principal source of sodium. However, it is also found in vegetables and muscle meats. Celery is particularly rich in sodium. A lack of sodium could result in muscle cramps, heat stroke, stomach and intestinal gas, weight loss, and muscle shrinkage. It favors the formation of saliva, gastric juice, enzymes, and other intestinal juices.

Sodium is also found in seafood, poultry, beets, chard, and dandelion greens. Other herbs include devil's bit scabious, meadowsweet, mistletoe, nettle leaves, cleavers, rest harrow, raspberry leaves, alfalfa, fennel seed, scarlet pimpernel, dandelion, black willow bark, and parsley.

The eighth mineral is *potassium.* It is important for body growth. Like sodium, it functions as a balancer, for sodium and potassium are needed in combination to help the body cells absorb nourishment from the bloodstream. It also assists in ridding the cells of waste matter. Dark and blackstrap molasses, dulse, kelp, leafy green vegetables, whole grains, fruits, and almonds are good sources of potassium. Other sources include American centaury, walnut leaves, mistletoe, chamomile flowers, yarrow, plantain leaves, scarlet pimpernel, alfalfa, eyebright, coltsfoot, birch bark, nettle leaves, couch grass, dandelion, calamus, sanicle, oak bark, parsley, watercress, primrose flowers, peppermint, and mountain mint. One of the richest sources of potassium is the banana.

A deficiency of potassium will cause constipation, nervous disorders, insomnia, slow and irregular heartbeat, and muscle damage. It sometimes causes the bones to become brittle and the kidneys to enlarge.

The ninth mineral is *magnesium,* which is necessary to maintain mineral balance in the body in hot weather and to promote sleep. It is an aid in digestion and in the elimination of foods. The best source of magnesium is found in figs, lemons, grapefruit, corn, brown rice, almonds, oil rich nuts and seeds, apples, and celery. Other sources are meadowsweet, rest harrow, toadflax, alfalfa, broom tops, black willow, walnut leaves, mistletoe, mullein leaves, silverweed, carrot leaves, primrose, and parsley.

About seventy percent of the magnesium found in the body is in the bones. The rest is in the soft tissues and blood. In blood, calcium needs about 5 percent magnesium to carry on its essential function. A lack of magnesium will often cause irritability, unhappiness, and interfere with normal sleep. In addition to a high vegetable diet, a pinch of epsom salts in a glass of water, once a week, can supply the magnesium you need.

The tenth mineral is *manganese.* This mineral gives strength to the tissues and bones and protects the inner lining of the heart and blood vessels. It works closely with the B-complex vitamins to overcome laziness, sterility, and marital weakness. It also combines with phosphorus to build strong bones. It is necessary to human growth and health, and is a good activator of the enzymes in our bodies.

Manganese is an essential element and makes tendons and muscles strong and elastic. Extra amounts may be helpful if you've had an accident and "pulled" a muscle.

If you grow some of your own vegetables, put a little kelp on your soil to replenish the manganese. Bone meal may also be used very sparingly.

Green, leafy vegetables, beans (green or dry), beets and beet leaf, egg yolks, natural unmilled grains, all supply a sufficient quantity of manganese unless you have an abnormal need. Other sources include parsley, lettuce, alfalfa, and spinach.

The eleventh mineral is *fluorine,* which helps build bones and tooth enamel and establishes the resistance of the body to disease and sickness. This is the natural fluorine which I am speaking about here, and it is found in many of the foods already named under the categories of the other minerals. It is said that when an excess is taken into the body, there is an adverse reaction upon internal organs, and there will be a weakening of the bone structure of the body. Additional sources of fluorine include watercress, beets, garlic, and spinach.

The twelfth category of minerals includes *carbon, hydrogen, oxygen,* and *nitrogen.* Of all the elements that go to make up the cells of the human body, it is said that these minerals are by far the most abundant, as they are found in all organic foods.

Few people ever realize the importance of these particular minerals because they seem so commonplace among the forty-four beneficial trace minerals which assist in the body structure of man.

The thirteenth mineral is *sulfur,* known as nature's beauty mineral, for it keeps the hair glossy, the complexion smooth and youthful. It also invigorates the bloodstream and makes it resistant to bacterial infection. It works on the liver to secrete bile, maintains an overall body balance, and influences the health of the brain tissues. The foods which contain sulfur are fish, eggs, cabbage, lean beef, dried beans, Brussels sprouts, and many of the leafy vegetables. Other sources are silverweed, nettle leaves, coltsfoot, calamus, broom tops, rest harrow, scarlet pimpernel, shepherd's purse, eyebright, plantain, meadowsweet, scouring rush, and mullein.

The greatest sources of sulfur are the proteins, the amino acids that have a sulfur link in the molecule. They must not be overheated as this liberates the sulfur and it becomes elemental and cannot be used by the body to build essential tissue. If you eat beans (dry beans), soak them overnight, let them sprout a few hours, and then cook slowly below the boiling point. You must use fresh beans — one year old or younger — to prepare them this way. When cooking eggs, use a thermal-controlled pan. Cook over 170 degrees, but under 200 degrees, and you'll be surprised how well they digest and how much better they taste.

The fourteenth mineral is *silicon,* responsible for keeping the skin firm, the body filled with vitality, the eyes bright and cheerful. It is found in the hair, muscles, nails, cellular walls, and connective tissues. It joins with other minerals to create tooth enamel and build strong bones. It is also said to be a builder of resistance to tuberculosis.

The food sources which are best for silicon are horsetail grass, buckwheat, corn, nuts, tomatoes, liver, lentils, and grains. Other sources include dandelion, spinach, strawberries, leek, horsetails, scouring rush, couch grass, knotgrass, and gravel plant.

The fifteenth mineral is *zinc,* a constituent of insulin and important to male reproductivity. It is used by the pancreas to store glycogen, an energy producing substance for the body. It combines with phosphorus to aid in respiration and in sparking vitamin action. It helps in tissue respiration, the intake of oxygen, and the expulsion of carbon dioxide and toxic wastes. Insulin is dependent upon zinc for functioning. The lack of insulin in the body leads to diabetes. Zinc helps food become absorbed through the intestinal walls and is part of the stomach enzymes. It assists in the manufacture of male hormones and connects with carbohydrates and energy.

There are many more known minerals, which influence our health and personality, but the fifteen shown here are the ones found in greatest abundance, and are very essential for good health and maintaining the body at a top efficiency level. Each of them needs the other minerals, for together they assist vitamins, proteins, amino acids, enzymes, carbohydrates, fats, sugars, and other necessary elements in the body.

Since most foods are deficient in essential minerals and vitamins due to poor soil and unfavorable marketing conditions, it is almost necessary to supplement the diet with natural mineral and vitamin supplements. There are a good many brands of natural minerals and vitamins on the market which can be recommended by physicians and health authorities.

It is important to be well informed on health matters. For example there is much misinformation regarding high blood pressure.

High blood pressure is caused by blood vessels which have lost their elasticity. They can no longer stretch and contract with each heartbeat. There are internal valves in the vessels carrying blood away from the heart. They open when the heart contracts and close after the contraction. It is this action which causes the blood to flow through the miles of blood vessels. The heart itself only forces the blood a short distance. It's this expansion and contraction, the closing and opening of valves, that moves the blood the many miles it must travel to supply the billions of cells with food and oxygen and carry away the wastes.

Anything that affects the elasticity of the blood vessels makes the heart work harder and causes high blood pressure.

The culprits which harden the arteries, causing a loss of elasticity, are:

1. Sugars which form triglycerides.
2. Fats which produce cholesterol.
3. Imbalance of salts.

Cholesterol comes from saturated fats, such as animal fats, hydrogenated fats (cooking oil/margarine), and the consumption of high carbohydrates with heavy proteins together at the same meal. We consume imbalanced salts when we use too much

sodium chloride (table salt) and do not have the beneficial trace minerals in our diet to balance it.

The popular low-salt or no-salt diet may not be for
everyone. Every chemical action that takes place in
your body (and there are over 10,000 such processes
going on) all take place in a solution of salt. If you
have dry or itchy skin, if you are light-headed and
dizzy, if you fatigue easily, etc., you probably lack
not only salt (table salt), but the related minerals —
potassium, calcium, phosphorus — and the other
essential factors which are found in seawater.

A lack of salt can cause a cellular sodium/potas-
sium imbalance that many believe can cause headache, chronic fatigue, and a predisposition to cellular
acidosis — a breeding ground for cancer and diabetes.

It is not that people are getting too much salt. It is
that their salt intake is out of balance because they
lack the potassium and trace minerals to make the
salt work for them. Seawater and seaweed (dulse)
supply these elements in abundance. Seawater can
usually be found in health food stores. The body's
need for seawater is quite meager — one-half to one
teaspoonful per day will generally be sufficient.

The survey of the means by which the separation
of Soul from the bondage of the body is accomplished would be far from complete if we did not take
up the Orphic and Eleusinian mysteries. Nectar, the
drink of the Olympian gods, was an infallible means
of initiation into the mysteries of the beyond by the
automatic release of Soul from bodily bondage.

Next we find the initiated Brahmans, the priests of
the Hindu religion, using what is known as the soma

44

drink. This was similar to the Greek nectar quaffed by the gods of Olympia. The cup of *Kykeon,* which was drunk at the initiation into the Eleusinian mysteries, was similar to both the Hindu and Greek god drinks.

He who would drink it easily reached the Brahma, the plane of splendor. The soma drink known to the Europeans was not the same as the one the Asiatics knew. Only the initiated can taste the real soma, and even the kings and rajas, when performing the sacrificial rites, received a substitute.

It is true that the priests of the present day orders have lost the secret of the true soma drink. It cannot be found in the rituals or the secret books anymore, nor through oral information. The true followers of the Vedic religion are now deceased, and the soma drink commemorated in the Hindu pantheon, which was called the King-soma, is gone, too. Whoever drank the King-soma participated in the heavenly kingdom. He became filled with the Holy Spirit and was purified of his sins.

The soma made a new man of the initiate; he was reborn and transformed, and his spiritual nature overcame the physical. It bestowed the divine power of inspiration and developed the clairvoyant faculty to the utmost. According to the esoteric explanation, the soma was a plant, but at the same time, it was an angel. It forcibly connected the initiate with the inner, a higher part of himself, and thus united by the power of the magic drink, he soared above the physical nature and participated in the beatitude and ineffable glories of heaven while still living on earth.

The soma drink was derived from a true plant which the priests used in the ancient rituals to separate Soul from the body during initiations in the mystery cults. We believe this to be frankincense, which was used in the ancient days for religious rituals, and if used as an incense, it was believed to bring the mind to devotion, producing a detached state of separation of Soul and body. It is said that the herb, which is a gum resin from various trees, was heated until it became a liquid, then mixed with honey and goat's milk. This became a powerful drink which would give the initiate the first step on the path of separation of Soul from the body.

The ECK Masters never used this sort of assistance for their chelas, because they felt that it was better to learn how to separate Soul and body with a clear consciousness. Nature has designed man to leave his physical body at will, transcend to higher planes, then return to the body. The Living ECK Master helps each aspirant or disciple of Eckankar personally, and each chela receives practical experience, however little. It may be during his initial experience with the Spiritual Exercises of ECK, or later. The person who is competent to give man this personal experience of withdrawal or separation from the body temporarily, and who can put him on the way to the higher spiritual realms, is the Living ECK Master, the Mahanta, the Vi-Guru.

The enzymes are delicate life-like substances found in all living cells, whether vegetable or animal. Their presence and strength can be determined only by means of refined tests. They consist primarily of an amino acid, a mineral, and vitamin-like substance, woven together. Enzymes act as catalysts for

46

chemical reactions in the body such as the breakup of other proteins, fats, starches, etc. There is practically no function carried on by the body that does not use enzymes. If a name of a substance or chemical name ends in ase, ine, or sin, often it is an enzyme.

One function of the enzyme is to aid in the digestion of food. They do this by accelerating specific chemical transformations in the digestion of foods. These specialized protein catalysts regulate the speed of the many chemical reactions involved in the metabolism of living organisms. The word *enzyme* is derived from the Greek word meaning "leavened."

Enzymes are classified into several broad categories, such as hydrolytic, oxidizing, and reducing, depending upon the type of reaction which they control. Nature puts enzymes into all foods together with vitamins, minerals, fats, proteins, carbohydrates, and water. However, all this food is completely indigestible until enzymes work on it and break down complex foods into simpler substances, which the bloodstream can then absorb. In addition, each enzyme must have a coenzyme, such as a vitamin or a mineral, before it can function.

There is an enzyme to help build phosphorus into bone and nerve tissues in the body. Another enzyme helps fix iron in the red blood cells. Enzymes can change protein into fat or sugar. Enzymes change carbohydrates into fat and enzymes change fats into carbohydrates.

Some enzymes, such as pepsin and trysin, which bring about the digestion of meat, control a great many different reactions, while others such as urease, which controls urea decomposition, are extremely specific and may accelerate only one reaction.

Enzymes perform in a few minutes chemical transformations which would be impossible without them. Without the help of enzymes we could stuff ourselves with herbs and foods but literally starve to death. The length of the life of enzymes depends upon temperature. When enzymes are subjected to boiling temperatures for even a few minutes, they are completely destroyed. Boiling potatoes, meats, or leafy vegetables in water often causes complete destruction of the enzymes contained therein.

Enzymes in the dormant state are found usually as dry seeds, and are able to retain their activity for hundreds of years. They have been found in the Egyptian mummies, which are over three thousand years old, in rice several hundred years old, and in the flesh of ancient mammoths found frozen in the Arctic regions. These mammoths are said to be over fifty thousand years old and still well-preserved. Enzymes can be preserved indefinitely when dried to a powder at blood heat or by extreme cold.

Enzymes can be extraordinarily efficient. When activated by hydrochloric acid, which is produced by the stomach from salt and acid (vinegar, etc.), one ounce of pepsin can digest nearly two tons of egg white. Notice on the label of a bottle of a digestive aid, it will mention pepsin 1/3000 or 1/15000, and list only a very small amount of it in that dilution. A tablet may only contain five or ten micrograms of diluted pepsin.

Sun-ripened fruits and vegetables are rich in enzymes. The sun causes enzymes to function, as they need warmth and moisture. But there is a difference between the sun warmth and the process of cooking. Therefore, in the manufacturing and cooking of foods, many enzymes are lost, which lowers the food value, and extra work is thrown upon the glands and organs: the liver, colon, stomach, intestines, kidneys, etc.

As each of us grows older, the quota of enzymes in the body gradually diminishes, and eventually, we die. This means that we are as old as our enzymes. The longevity of the ECK Masters is partly due to the fact that they have learned to control the enzymes in their physical bodies. But the average person can keep his body functioning well under general conditions, as long as he has sufficient enzymes to digest the foods that he eats.

In order to have less wear on the body and to save it from aging too fast, one can try to take into his body the exogenous enzymes—those enzymes which are derived from raw foods. It is these uncooked, unprocessed foods which give the body the exogenous enzymes. The more enzymes consumed in the raw and uncooked foods, the fewer the body will have to manufacture on its own.

Knowledge about enzymes proves the relationship between good health and long life of the ECK Masters. Their diet, which consists largely of natural uncooked foods, includes fruits and vegetables, mostly in an unaltered state from the soil to their mouths.

One of the best enzymes that a person can find for his health is contained in pineapple. This is the reason the peoples of the South Sea Islands remained in

49

such general good health before the coming of the white man. The papaya also ranks high in enzymes. Either one or the other should be eaten with every meal if possible, as both are high in enzymes which greatly aid the digestion.

Enzyme-rich foods that may be added to our diet are: all raw vegetables and fruits, raw seeds, sunflower seeds, sesame, flax, chia, all nuts if raw and not roasted, dry herbs sprinkled over foods and salads, and raw vegetable/fruit juices (diluted with one-third water). Canned foods do not contain enzymes, nor do foods that are processed, baked, cooked, smoked, pickled, etc. It is best to keep your diet simple and ideally to cook no more than about twenty percent of the food eaten.

Some of the other foods which may be added to our diet to help with the intake of minerals, proteins, vitamins, enzymes, and other essential ingredients for good health are: almonds, coconuts, pecans, walnuts, hazelnuts, lecithin, honey, wheat germ, brewer's yeast, yogurt, buttermilk, fish, kidneys, liver, apricots, pumpkins, sesame, apples, eggs, cottage cheese and sun-ripened dried fruits. These are not all, of course, only a few to get you started on the right path to better health and longevity.

3

The Herbs That Give Life
for the Vital Powers

Half of the population of the United States suffers from some form of chronic disease, and only a small percentage of all Americans are free from any kind of physical ailment or defect, according to the report of the U.S. Special Commission on the Nation's Health given to the president in December, 1964.

We have more mental hospitals and sanatoriums, more psychiatrists and psychoanalysts than any country in the world, but it has been estimated that one out of every ten Americans may spend some part of his life in a mental institution.

Where did man drop the natural path to health through herbs, plants, minerals, and vitamins and begin on the path of chemistry for his health? Sometime after the end of the Middle Ages and the beginning of this modern age, Lavoisier, Pasteur, Harvey, Cesalpino, Schleiden, and others might have taken the wrong turn on the path to good health.

Nature is the destroyer of all living organisms, and there is not much man can do about it, despite all his wonderful advances in a science that is praised as being the greatest in all history. Soul is immortal, but man as the body will be born, live, and die like everything else in the world.

Sir Thomas Browne, a physician who lived in England, made the statement, "Death is the only cure to every problem of man, but everybody that I know seems to be fighting off the cure." In time all must die. It is only the ECK Masters who have the secrets for longevity, and it is hardly thinkable that they are going to give out their knowledge to the masses of the world.

The world is already overpopulated and nature always has a way of taking care of this phenomenon whenever it takes place on earth. If a major war does not reduce the population of the human race so others might live, then a vast catastrophe takes place and large masses of people are suddenly taken out of their bodies. This is why the Living ECK Master is now striving so hard to arouse Souls to get out of their bodies naturally and return to the higher worlds so they will not have to be reincarnated into this world where a major cataclysm is going to take place.

However, we find a need for living in better health in the present moment. There is a remedy through herbs, plants, diet, moderate fasting, and the philosophy of Eckankar. You may call it the ECK diet, for through it you can find your way to health once more.

One must begin an independent study at the very roots of his nutritional necessities. He must seek to learn the physical, chemical, and biological origin of his body. He should put aside all psychological and spiritual questions until later. He begins with the theory and practice of nutrition, of which the first principles are: (1) Every living thing in the organic world exists through the intake of air, water, food, and rest by sleep; and (2) anything that has life and is deprived of air, water, food, or rest by sleep will soon die.

The principle for man to note here is that food is to be eaten for the survival of the body. Survival is also the concern of the most spiritual of mankind, for even those spiritual giants who have walked the earth ate food, breathed air, and drank water. The body is a transformation of food; therefore, eating is being.

In Atlantis, flowers, cereals — both wild and cultivated — grew in great abundance and variety, including one fruit which is known to have had a hard rind and to have provided both meat and ointment. This was the coconut, for Atlantis was in a semitropical zone and many of the crops raised were warm-climate plants. The Atlanteans also had orchards. Most of their cereal crops were wheat, oats, barley, rye, and maize. Their meats were produced from domesticated animals, especially raised for the purpose of feeding the massive population of Atlantis.

During my incarnations in Atlantis, which are now ancient memories, the people were tall, fair-haired, with good figures and blue eyes. Those inhabitants of Lemuria, in the area of what is now the Pacific Ocean, as I remember, were fairly tall, slender, with dark olive skins and brown or black eyes and hair.

The people of both continents were great fish eaters. They were more inclined to eat fish and fowl rather than beef or pork, and their diet included fruits, vegetables, herbs, and cereals, especially wheat.

They ate a great deal of fresh fruit, flat wheat wafers, buck loin, fish, chicken, or birds of any nature which the professional hunters would trap by the scores and sell to the open-air markets in the large public squares of the many vast cities on Atlantis. Most of their meats, however, were roasted. They never ate fried meat because it was considered to be bad for the stomach.

The tradition and policy of the Atlanteans about meat was that it was well to eat it, but not as a staple diet. Animal flesh contained, so they believed, certain properties which were of value when taken with discretion. But eaten frequently, and in too large a quantity, meat would coarsen the body and lead to many of the internal complaints which are so prevalent among the races of the world today.

A liquid drink was made from the coconut milk which was an opaque, green-yellow color. It was a fruit juice diluted with coconut milk and water, mixed with limes and granadillas.

They also had a cordial to aid the digestion. It was a dark, sticky, green liqueur, not unlike Chartreuse. It was flavored with flowers and herbs and was highly alcoholic. The taste was fiery and would cause a warm glow in the stomach and body when swallowed.

The people of Atlantis bathed in hot springs with an oil that would lather. These springs were housed in stone buildings similar to the Roman baths. Mixed bathing was quite popular and few considered this more than a social gathering of families who would visit while they washed, rested, bathed, and sunned themselves. Most of them wore light clothes similar to Roman togas and gowns because the weather was mild.

Whenever they wished to eat, especially the peasant class, they would gather fresh fruit which was in season and net a fish in the lake or river and cook it. All waste products were disposed of by burying in the soil. They tapped the sunlight for many things — for example, heating water in containers which would be under a sort of glass similar to our ultraviolet ray.

The Atlanteans had thirty thousand years in which to develop their civilization, so there is little wonder that it was greater than anything we find on earth today. They were able to control all the world by force of arms and political means, as most of it was colonized by the Atlanteans. When modern man is able to fully explore the other planets there will be found ruins of a civilization which cannot be explained. It will be the remains of colonies which the Atlanteans settled upon these planets for trade purposes and because their homeland was becoming overcrowded. These colonies eventually died after Atlantis sank beneath the waves centuries ago.

The Atlanteans grew cereals in abundance, as well as radishes, carrots, turnips, lettuce, dwarf beans, peas, potatoes, broccoli, cabbage, and artichokes. There were also many other plants whose names would not be at all familiar to the reader, such as the atoge, which was a type of yellow corn, and the vladige, a type of sweet potato.

Many of their herbal formulas consisted of tonics, aromatics, laxatives, purgatives, and antispasmodics. Herbs, seeds, roots, and plants accomplished much for the general health of the Atlantean nation. Among those which were used most in the general curative formulas were celery, musk root, vervain, jasmine, coriander, navel wort, wild poppy, purslane, maidenhair, valerian, anemone, endive, myrtle, mandrake, cloves, cinnamon, cardamom, and hemlock.

The Living ECK Master (known as Supaku) of one of the high periods of the civilization of Atlantis helped to compile a number of the herbs, roots, seeds, flowers, and plants which were researched in the government health laboratories. Some of these are described below:

Angelica is a domestic herb which was used to give added strength when the body needed an extra push. The Atlanteans used this for their common foot soldiers in battle. It was also used as a stomach medicine for gas and as a mild diaphoretic.

Anise is another plant that was used by the Atlanteans. The oil was used as a base for liquors, and, as today, in preparations for pectoral troubles arising from colds, coughs, etc. Anise was also used as a medicine for the relief of intestinal gases caused by meals consisting of too much pork and beef.

Basil, another herb of the mint family, was used a great deal by the Atlanteans. It is a sweet herb characterized by a pleasant smell and taste. It was used for seasoning and flavoring foods, and for intestinal gases and mild nervous disorders. It is still being used for the same purposes in modern times.

Chamomile, a plant of the aster family, was often used by the Atlanteans. It has strong scented foliage and flower heads which contain a bitter medicinal principle. It is used as an antispasmodic, stomachic, and as a perspiration-producing ingredient for breaking fevers. It is used for nervous conditions of the body, poultices for allaying pain, and when made as a tea, is effective as a sedative. It also makes a good hair shampoo lotion.

Comfrey is a very useful herb, which is now considered by the U.S. government and English authorities to be a cancer proliferator. It should only be used outside the body as a poultice or dressing. In those ancient times it was described by a word which we would call "knitbone." It was used mainly as a poultice for diseased and fractured bones.

The common *dandelion* is another plant which the Atlanteans made use of for kidney and liver disorders. They also used its root for roasting and making a drink similar to coffee.

Garlic was the miracle herb of the day in those ancient times, as it is in this modern era. It was used to break fevers, as a diuretic, and as a healing agent for wounds both inner and outer. It was made into a syrup with honey and used by those who had common colds and respiratory diseases, just as it is today.

The Atlanteans used ground ivy as an astringent, diuretic, and tonic for kidney diseases and for indigestion. Also, horehound was a popular herbal

57

expectorant. Then there was hyssop, which they used for healing wounds, for coughs, and lung complaints; and sweet marjoram, pot marjoram, and mint for nausea, sickness, and children's illnesses. They used nettles, parsley, rosemary, rue, tansy, thyme, wormwood, mugwort, valerian, satyrion as well as a dozen others which are unknown today.

I have used the modern terms for these herbs, because the Atlantean names for each probably could not be pronounced because of the difference between the Atlantean languages and English. But we do know that apricots were a staple food for the Atlanteans. They used them in everything, and they carried them as a dried food for long voyages in ships that sailed the seas and in interplanetary spaceships.

We know that all foods have a vegetal origin. Animals could not exist without the vegetal. The human body cannot digest inorganic substances. It cannot manufacture carbohydrates, fats, or minerals from inorganic substances. The synthesis of inorganic substances is a vegetal function, a process called autotropism. This is a phenomenon performed by the vegetable kingdom in which inorganic elements are absorbed and converted into organic foods — a miracle of composition and creation produced by the interworking forces of nature.

Whether it is worth man's efforts to be a meat eater is still a moot question. A few persons have demonstrated the value of giving up meat if one is going to have spiritual unfoldment, and others have demonstrated that meat eating has little influence on whether a person gets spiritual unfoldment or not.

However, we first take up the vegetable kingdom as an individual factor in the eating process for health in man. The vegetable kingdom works ceaselessly to produce the leaves, grains, tubers, and fruits which feed fleshly organisms, such as animals and man. The vegetable is mother to the animal and human species. These leaves, grains, tubers, and fruits are transformed into animal tissue by the process of digestion and assimilation.

Man is the child of the vegetal mother, so say some people who are close students of herbs, plants, and flowers. Without vegetable life, so they claim, no animal or human life could survive on earth. This is accepted, of course, for we are utterly dependent, directly or indirectly, upon vegetable and fruit produce for our physical survival. The hemoglobin of the blood cells is derived from chlorophyl. All vegetal foods are the virgin materials for the maintenance and construction of body tissues, so this means we must have vegetables as our basic food. This is a biological and fundamental law.

Many people are vegetarians for this reason, yet the law does not apply to all people, as stated before, for there are many who simply cannot be vegetarians because of something in their physical systems which will not allow it.

Too many of those who believe that the chemistry of people is uniform learn in the long run that what one thinks is right about dieting can be all wrong for another. No two people can follow the same diet for many reasons. One may be karmic conditions, another could be the environmental conditions learned at mother's knee. Physical heredity and astrological influences may also contribute to individual differences.

No two people have the same reaction to a given food intake. Whereas one person can be a good vegetarian, another would become ill if put on such a diet for any length of time. Some ECK Masters, the Adepts of the Ancient Order of Vairagi, have been meat eaters, not heavily, of course, but they ate fish and fowl. Others within the order have been pure vegetarians. The ECK Masters are above the body consciousness and cannot be affected by what is put in their bodies in the way of food. Naturally, none of them drink or smoke.

The idea of vegetarianism is an old one. Traditionally, it has been linked with the spiritual growth of man via the Oriental religions. Millions in India, China, Japan, and other countries of the Far East have for centuries followed the vegetarian diet. Vegetarianism started in the ancient days when the domestic animal was a scarce item and the *Laws of Manu,* which possibly appeared as the law book which codified the ancient Hindu law, said that the killing of the cow was a religious taboo.

This law book also included mythology, cosmogony, metaphysical doctrines, techniques of government, duties of the various castes, and the doctrines of immortality and transmigration of Soul.

There was a judge in India during these ancient times who tried to help the poor by decreeing that killing a cow was a violation of civil law (in order to protect the family's supply of dairy products). Families in those early days had to depend upon the cow's milk, butter, and cheese as their main source of food.

If a neighbor or a thief stole the cow and butchered it for meat, the family was left destitute.

The law did not work very well, so the civil authorities decided that it would be better to incorporate it into the *Laws of Manu* as sacred law to be enforced by the priestcraft. Hence vegetarianism became a necessity with millions of the poor in India, a part of the religious tradition. To this day the cow is sacred in India, and much of the population will not eat meat because of this. Vegetarianism has become a fixed idea in the minds of many of the religious teachers, who claim that only the vegetarians shall have spiritual enlightenment.

Other countries such as China, Japan, and the nations of Southeast Asia also have their traditions of vegetarianism, but this has remained more out of necessity, because of the lack of domestic animals for human consumption.

During primitive times there was not enough food to supply the teeming population, so a majority of people in the Asian countries became vegetarians. However, we find today that the people on a whole are not as healthy in these countries. They are small in stature and are generally in bad health with shorter life spans.

In the beginning, we find that the ECK (positive or God) foods and the Kal (negative) foods are just opposite in nature. The Kal is always opposite to, and antagonistic to, the ECK, yet it cannot exist without its superior which is the ECK. In this relativistic material world, the ECK is antithetical and opposite to the Kal. Happiness is the opposite of sadness, and beauty is the opposite of ugliness. Each thing within this universe is supported, animated, maintained, and is in opposition to its opposite. This is the great Law of the SUGMAD, which is the order of the universe. It is the very simple yet profound law which rules our life in this relative world as distinguished from the true world of Spirit, that which is absolute, infinite, and eternal.

If one has violated this great law of the universe, he could die prematurely because of illness or accident. The ECK is tolerant and forgiving to the very end. But if we violate Its laws, while living in this world of matter, energy, space, and time, we must pay the penalty. There is no excuse for being ignorant of the law. If we are ill, it is only meant to be a warning, an alarm signal, and not a punishment. Too many ignore this divine alarm signal and go to the drugstore to find a pain-relieving drug on the shelf. The use of drugs or other drastic means to heal, such as patent medicines and other methods, only serves to destroy the delicate alarm signals.

There are two ways that drugs are harmful to the body—one is that drugs will only arrest the progress of a disease, but seldom cure it; second, that drugs are generally devoid of morality and spirituality, having been developed at any cost and method to destroy the symptoms of disease. Drugs often create more serious illness and disease in future generations by arresting a malady at its present stage of progress within the body.

The essential aim of ECK is to lead man to infinite freedom, absolute justice, and eternal happiness by the means of Soul Travel. We keep running into problems with this aim of Eckankar, because most people want to make a garbage pail of their bodies and regard spirituality as something separate from their health.

This is not true, for health has a bearing upon the spiritual development of each individual, whether he knows it or not. That is, the state of the body has an influence upon the mind, and the mind, in turn, can affect the spiritual side of those not yet trained in the spiritual arts of Soul Travel. When one has reached a certain stage of spiritual unfoldment, he will have the self-discipline so that nothing can affect him. This is known as the *vairag,* or the true detachment from the material world. But at the stage of spiritual unfoldment that most people have reached at the present time, few have any discipline whatsoever.

A diseased or sick body has a direct influence upon the non-disciplined person and will affect his mental attitude as well as his food intake. Therefore, the man seeking spiritual enlightenment will become acquainted with herbs, minerals, plants, and flowers as a means of improving his health. Then he can concentrate on his spiritual unfoldment, instead of a body which reflects illness and pain.

The knowledge of nutrition that we find in the ECK knowledge of herbs offers much toward the curing of some basic illnesses in the individual. There are several approaches to health which should be of interest. First is the symptomatic remedy, which is a palliative means of removing symptoms. Second is the preventive remedy, which arrests an illness or keeps it from happening. Third is the study of the means of attaining better physical, mental, and spiritual health. Fourth is the Kal (negative) means of trying to keep the body healthy by narcotics or similar drugs. Fifth, the social and educational means, which establishes health institutions for the public at large. Sixth, the remedy of mental and philosophical means, directed to the plane of thought and self-help (i.e. certain forms of yoga and other spirito-materialistic philosophies which have to do with exercises of the mind and body). Last is the ECK (God or positive) method of finding health. Through Soul Travel, which lifts one above this physical plane of consciousness, one can see and repair whatever damage is done to the body and brain.

Those in Eckankar know that there are several methods of taking care of the physical health of the body and mind: by the intake of herbs, minerals, vitamins, fruits, vegetables, and flowers in the correct form; by prayer, which is seldom used by any ECK chela; by contemplation or the use of the Spiritual Exercises of ECK; and last, by Soul Travel itself. If one is praying, using meditation, or any of the esoteric methods of asking God for healing, he may be answered in different ways. First, his prayer might be answered on the physical level by someone indirectly suggesting that he use certain medications, herbs, remedies, or that he see a particular physician. The second way in which he might receive help is through the inner senses flashing a message for guidance in a certain direction. The third method is, of course, direct healing from the Living ECK Master or from other divine sources which render the healing possible.

To find the particular remedy that will eliminate the cause of an ailment for good is the purpose of the

ECK methods. The ECK remedy is the highest way, and, indeed, it is the simplest method, but the deepest in its philosophical foundation. Since the ultimate cause of every illness is a violation of the order of the universe through ignorance, few attack this cause and restore their health. The ECK way of restoring health is through patience, using the philosophy and education in the spiritual works of ECK in order to get the chela to know something about himself.

The ECK way is to show man how to release his own innate abilities so that he might successfully achieve good judgment, good health within this world, success at Soul Travel, and spiritual perfection leading to God-Realization.

It is true that faith has a great deal to do with the healing of the body and mind, but it is not everything. If faith could cure, then all those who make pilgrimages to Lourdes would be healed. Naturally, faith will heal some but, in a way, it might injure others who lack the understanding necessary for healing. Blind faith is often primitive, filled with superstitions, unguided, and misdirected.

It is said in the works of ECK that faith—that is, true faith—must insist upon the understanding of the divine cause of whatever life might be. This is, of course, an understanding of the laws of Karma, retribution and reincarnation. Thus, faith can be considered as knowledge, for without knowledge beyond the physical senses, there can be no true faith.

We find that most of us put blind faith in medicines. We hope that the health authorities will have enough knowledge to heal us or get rid of the cause of our illness. The use of medicine of itself requires blind faith. Who is man going to trust to help him get rid of all those causes of illness?

Those who follow the path of Eckankar, the Ancient Science of Soul Travel, know that it is best to put one's faith in the Living ECK Master, who is really the Mahanta, the living Divine Consciousness on earth, said to be symbolic of the ancient law that has prevailed over all life here in this world. This is known to all ECK chelas as the Tejas, the radiant principle, that law of God which is the practical philosophy of the ECK and the Kal. The ECK power may be called the centripetal wave which is always moving toward the center (that is, the Heavenly Kingdom), the Ocean of Love and Mercy. The Kal power is that wave which is said to be moving away from the center of life.

The ECK and Kal are at the same time in opposition and yet complementary to one another like day and night, summer and winter, man and woman. They are the fundamental opposites which destroy and unite to create everything that exists in the lower worlds.

Because in this world the ECK is always limited and relative, it means that the Kal, which is the lower world power, is also limited and relative. But here in this world they blend into each other like night and day. We find that nothing exists that is totally Kal or totally ECK in this world. It is either more Kal than ECK, or more ECK than Kal, so we think of them as being one or the other.

This is the dualism which we read so much about in the sacred scriptures of the world. In this world of relativity we find that the ECK inevitably changes

66

into the Kal and the Kal into the ECK. It is when we enter into the worlds of pure Spirit above the Atma, the Fifth, or Soul, Plane, that we find the absolute, eternal, and infinite.

We find that within this category of the ECK and Kal there are degrees of characteristics. The three fundamental characteristics are shape, weight, and color. We find that the ECK is not limited because It is the positive God force. Therefore, It will lack a shape, for It is a great wave which is collecting all Souls in the worlds of God and returning them to the great Ocean of Love and Mercy, from the negative pole to the highest of the worlds. It is like an ocean wave which feeds all life. It dominates all life in a weightless degree and in the pale colors which are pinks, oranges, high yellows, light greens, and sky blues.

Everything in the universe can be classified as either ECK or Kal without getting into any complications. Most products grown in the cooler climates are ECK, in comparison with those grown in the warm climates. The red fruits from the northern climates (for example, apples) are ECK foods; while those like the purple mango from the tropical countries are listed among the Kal foods.

Therefore, we find that the Kal is the heavier of the two forces for it dwells in the lower worlds. It makes the solidness which we call the soil and other forms of inorganic life. Many of the colors of Kal fruits, plants, and other organic foods are purple, dull orange, indigo, dark red, dark green, black, and heavy yellow.

We note that those who live in a temperate climate where the cooler weather is more prevalent are usually psychologically stronger than those races living in the tropics, because the former eat more ECK foods than the latter. Now we also find that the ECK foods are mildly sweet and pleasant tasting while the Kal foods are generally hot, pungent, sour, heavily sweet, bitter, and salty. This pertains only to the natural tastes and not to artificial flavors or those chemically treated.

Most ECK foods are red or yellow, generally pale in color. We even find this true of meats which are to be found on the butcher's counter (not frozen or canned meats). This also is true of fish, eggs, and dairy products. We find the following are ECK foods: pumpkins, carrots, yams, apples, cherries, strawberries, brown rice, oranges, all vegetables, cereals, fruits and plants of natural pale colors. These are strong in vitamins, minerals, and enzymes.

The Kal foods are generally the artificially prepared foods. They are the pastries, pies, and breads made from refined flours and hydrogenated fats, chocolate flavoring, candy, soft drinks, synthetic ice cream. Also foods with a natural dark coloring, like eggplant, mango, pimiento, red peppers or any other type of hot seasoning, watercress and dark red vegetables such as some beans.

One should add lots of seeds to his diet which are ECK in nature, such as pumpkin, sesame, almond, and other types of nuts (not salted nuts, but those that are raw or have been roasted only in pure oil). One should also add to the diet brewer's yeast, lecithin, and wheat germ. These products can be eaten with cottage cheese and salads or mixed in fruit juices and yogurt if one desires. Buttermilk can be included in the diet; and one should eat some meat, especially brains, kidney, and liver. These are generally good for the human system.

The essential factor in this nutrition discussion about the ECK and Kal food value is that there should be a proper proportion of each for the human body to have the right nourishment daily. Unless this is done, one will suffer from a lack of, for example, potassium, a Kal product necessary for the nourishment and feeding of the body system. Potassium must be properly balanced in the body with sodium, an ECK product, in order to feed the body properly.

However, we find that the best all around food product, which contains a perfect balance between the ECK and the Kal foods, is natural, unpolished brown rice. If one's environmental habits are broken or disturbed and meat cannot be eaten because of some body ailment, he can turn to natural, unpolished brown rice to give him most of the nourishment his body needs for good health.

4

The Magic of the Wonder Herbs

Anyone who raises questions about man's health and philosophical nature must be prepared to answer those who come swarming to him about their own issues of life, be it here in the physical body or the spiritual self.

Man's desire for better health leads him to begin to pinpoint those few herbs and minerals which can give him special help. The wonder herbs are not many, although we can say that every plant and herb is a gift of God to man. Therefore, we could really look at each as a wonder herb.

It may clarify matters if it is pointed out that all vegetables are herbs, regardless of whether they are called foods or medicines. Unless this is understood, it is quite useless to study herbs. Those chelas who assimilate and keep the fundamentals of herbology in mind will be more successful in attaining results.

A hundred years ago, all plants were divided into two major categories: Usable Herbs and Non-Usable

Herbs. The usable herbs were further divided into three sub-categories:
1. Pot Herbs — now called vegetables
2. Mild Herbs — those used for medicine and seasoning
3. Drastic Herbs — the poison, toxic, or corrosive herbs which we try to avoid.

The mild herbs were used for healing the sick. They were never intended to be used in ignorance.

Herbs vary greatly in their effectiveness. People taking herbs will react individually to the different herbs. So we find that there are two major considerations and sources of inconsistency in herbal treatment for each illness: 1) The individual himself and how he will respond to a given herb; 2) The herb and its effect on the particular individual.

No two people react exactly the same to any given herb; no herb will effect the same reaction in every person taking that herb. A combination of herbs may well affect a greater percentage of individuals in a positive manner. If a single herb works for you, then stay with it; if a single herb doesn't work for you, then you may wish to try a different herb or combination of herbs.

A few herbs have been designated as miracle herbs — for example, potato, pimiento, leptotaenia, kola nut, kelp, licorice, alfalfa, goldenseal, hawthorn, parsley, and the mint family. There are more, but these and a few others are to be taken up in this chapter and discussed at length.

Nature's process of healing is gradual and always seems terribly slow to those who are suffering or impatient. While herbs will assist, it is always God who does the healing. To give up the harmful indulgences requires self-discipline on the part of the sufferer. But it must be done. Habits that have injured the body in the past must be dropped. We find those who persevere in self-discipline and abide by the laws of Spirit will gain results in health of the body and mind. No man living in this material universe can go on disobeying the laws of this world and expect to have good health.

The herb *goldenseal* could be placed at the top of any "Ten Most Wanted Herbs" list. We mainly find it used among the Indian tribes of North America. They relied on it almost entirely for many of their medical needs. Not having the science of medicine as we do today, the North American natives had to depend wholly upon the plant and herb kingdom for their medicinal needs. This was natural, and much of their findings have been brought into our research laboratories so that we might understand just what the Indians had to help them keep their health under such primitive conditions.

Goldenseal grows in moist, rich woodlands in various parts of the United States, from Connecticut to the Gulf Coast, but it is most abundant in the south. It is a very expensive herb because of limited supplies due to difficulty in harvesting and distribution.

It is a small plant with a solitary rose-colored or whitish flower. The fruit, which looks much like a raspberry, is not edible, and the leaves are seldom used. The root is dark brown when first dug up. After being thoroughly washed and dried, it is powdered and has a greenish yellow tint.

The American Indians used this herb as a dye for cloth. It is thought that this dyeing action is responsible for goldenseal being such a good, selective antibiotic. The thought is that goldenseal dyes the harmful bacteria yellow, and the bacteria then lose the power to reproduce and die out. It is selective in that it does not appear to affect the beneficial coliform bacteria, lactobacillus.

Goldenseal is probably the most universal herb; it is said to help the whole body. With the exception of the pancreas, it benefits every organ of the body. It was believed to correct the cause of both dysentery and constipation, to aid digestion, to be a detoxifier, to toughen flabby tissues, heal wounds, and fight infections and fevers.

Even so, persistent, long-time use of this wonder herb is not recommended as it drains the body of B vitamins (B_1, B_6, B_{12}, etc). Its action stimulates the metabolism and will cause an increased demand for some of the B vitamins and vitamin C. So, if goldenseal is used more than five or six consecutive days, be sure to take extra B vitamins and vitamin C.

As a laxative, one-half teaspoon or one to two capsules of goldenseal can bring overnight relief. One capsule of goldenseal is helpful for a sour stomach; for indigestion or flatulence, one capsule two to three times a day; for fever, two capsules every ten hours; for infections of all kinds, one capsule three times a day for a general clearing in three days.

Goldenseal mixed with lard is said to be a fantastic healing cream — using coconut oil as a base is even better. This wonder cream can be used topically for burns, scalds, cuts, scrapes, scratches, blisters,

74

insect bites, and sores of all kinds; but it does stain, so be careful.

Boils and blood infections respond beautifully to a regimen of three capsules of goldenseal per day and one gallon of good water for two or three days. This makes a good blood cleanser for almost any kind of infection or toxic blood disorder.

It is reported that people have used goldenseal successfully for treating colds, flu, fever, constipation, indigestion, chills, rashes, sore throat, gum problems (put powder directly on "sores"), chancres, fever blisters, cystitis (bladder inflammation), liver and spleen infections and inflammations, boils, topically for sores, scratches, burns, rashes, insect bites, etc.

One caution about using goldenseal is that it stains skin and clothing and is difficult to remove. Do not apply goldenseal while wearing clothing which might be damaged by it.

If you wish to use goldenseal as a dye for cloth, thread, etc., here is the method:

1. Use one tablespoon of goldenseal powder to one quart of water.
2. Soak mixture at least twelve hours (overnight).
3. Bring mixture to a slow simmer for fifteen to twenty minutes.
4. Strain mixture while it's still hot.
5. Soak fabric in this hot solution for thirty minutes.
6. Add one-fourth cup vinegar and one tsp. alum and mix.
7. Heat and bring to a simmer. Stir.
8. Let stand until cool.

9. Remove fabric, rinse with cold, running water until water runs clear.
10. Sun dry the fabric.

Most fabrics will dye to a light burnt-orange color. This color can be changed to a lighter yellow color by reducing the amount of vinegar added and also adding table salt to the mixture.

One surprising wonder herb is the lowly, common tuber, the *potato*. Most people spend their lives eating potatoes either mashed, baked, boiled, or fried. Similarly, most people are not aware that this wonderful food can be used for healing. It is possible to treat a poison ivy and poison sumac rash with the pounded up leaves of the potato vine made into a paste to be topically applied to the affected area. This is then covered with a bandage of pounded straw on yellow dock leaves. This treatment could reduce the inflammation in twelve hours and heal completely in forty-eight!

A raw, mashed potato can be used to treat minor abrasions and wounds in minutes. It is also cooling for minor burns. Finely shredded, mixed with raw egg white, and carefully applied to the affected area, this potato mixture will allay the pain from minor burns, scaldings, and sunburn most effectively. Mild acid burns and also toxic-chemical eye injuries may respond favorably to a paste of raw, ground potato placed over the burned area and replaced every twenty minutes.

Drinking *fresh* potato juice can have miraculous effects. The raw potato contains very important enzymes and is a wonderful source of vitamin C.

Early sailors did not contract scurvy if their rations included raw potatoes. If they did come down with scurvy, they could overcome it by eating raw potatoes. Many people with highly toxic conditions could become normal by drinking potato juice.

A sore mouth, bad gums, sore throats, colds, croup, swollen glands, stomach ulcers, colon ulcers, bleeding bowels and bladder—all respond very quickly to the use of potato juice.

Potato juice should be drunk immediately after juicing as it loses its effectiveness very quickly; in fact, within fifteen minutes, it will have lost most of its effectiveness. CAUTION! *Use only red potatoes.* The russet (brown) baking potato contains an antiproteoletic enzyme which will inhibit the digestion of proteins and cause autointoxication, constipation, headache, stomach cramps, etc. The sprouts of all potatoes contain a toxic substance, solanine, and so should never be eaten. The green color that potatoes acquire from having grown partially out of the ground or having been on display for several days in the market under fluorescent lighting also contain this toxic alkaloid. Luckily, cooking will destroy it. If you must use green potatoes, be sure to cook them well; it is best to remove all the green portions as, even when well cooked, they impart a bitter, off-flavor to the potato.

It is said that to heal peptic ulcers, you should drink three cupfuls of *freshly* produced potato juice daily. Eat only vegetables that are cooked by the "stir fry" method of cooking in a small amount of water—one or two tablespoons per quart. Eat nothing else! The second day you should experience a subsiding of pain; by the fifth day (unless the ulcer is very large) you should have a healed ulcer and be able to return to carefully eating other foods and beverages — in moderation, of course.

The potato is also an excellent, almost miraculous, beauty pack — far superior to commercial products containing expensive and exotic ingredients, including perfume oils to add to the mystique. Whenever fresh potato juice is made, a by-product of pulp and potato starch is also produced. This by-product of white starch can be spread on the skin of the face and rubbed into those areas where the skin is coarse, flaky, or a problem area. Allow the paste to remain on the skin for fifteen minutes, and then rinse off with cool water. You'll be amazed at the soft, beautiful skin engendered by this process. This method has been used on harsh, red, rough "dishpan" hands and within one week's time, the hands are much improved. If the skin is extremely cracked and dry, add a cup of raisins to the potato pulp and starch (of course you have already drunk the fresh potato juice) and blend for a few seconds. Apply this mixture to the skin, allow it to remain for fifteen minutes, and then rinse off in cool water. You'll be truly amazed at the results.

The third wonder herb is the *pimiento* (a sweet pepper), profusely grown in northern Italy. Originally, peppers came from the Amazon.

There are basically three kinds of peppers in the sweet and hot varieties:

1. Cayenne pepper. It is long and rather small in diameter (about 1 1/4 inches) and about eight inches in length. It is the cheapest and is often quite hot. Also called the chili pepper.

2. The red bell pepper. Generally, it is a sweet, mild pepper often grown in gardens. This is the familiar, bell-shaped (wide at the top and wide at the bottom) pepper having several longitudinal ridges or creases from top to bottom.

3. The pimiento variety. This is a heart-shaped pepper, wide at the top and gently tapering to a rather pointed bottom. It is about three-fourths as wide at the top as it is in length. The meat of the pimiento is crisp and thick, and the flavor can be slightly hot, mellow, or mildly sweet.

Throughout the world, there are groups of people who live very long lives — many are over 100 years old. There are such groups in Russia, in China, in the Himalayas, and in the Yucatan Peninsula; however, it was in northern Italy that the key was found to these various people's longevity. Each of these groups had a common herb usage in their diets — each used a lot of pimiento paprika on an almost daily basis. When grown, the green pimiento is allowed to ripen to a rich, ruby-like red; it is then dried and *stone* ground to form a thick powder. This powder is then mixed with hot water and other herbs or natural products to make a soup similar in color and consistency to our tomato soup. Sometimes cracked or ground seeds and/or nutmeats, as well as pimiento, are added to wheat cakes and other dishes of varying kinds. Most of the adults appear to eat about two tablespoonfuls of pimiento each day in one food or another.

In analyzing this miracle food (herb), we find that it contains the richest sources of the substances the body utilizes to manufacture connective tissue (collagen): vitamin C, vitamin A, calcium, phosphorus, zinc, chromium, amino acids, flavones, citrines, and bioflavonoids. It also contains the hormones necessary to maintain the heart. It would be hard to find a more perfect food supplement for building a strong body and a strong heart.

By adding to this miracle herb some saguaro cactus berries, which clean the sugar and triglycerides out of the blood vessels, some cinnamon bark to increase the circulation and strengthen the capillary system, and hawthorn berries to control blood pressure, you can produce a formula which is ideal for the heart and circulatory system. It is said that a person is really only as old as his arteries. People have overcome angina pectoris and high blood pressure, arteries have been cleared out and strengthened, and a general feeling of well-being restored by these simple but beautiful herbs.

Your body is made from and maintained by food, and only proper food can rebuild damaged tissues. Medicines cannot build, they often only serve to whip a tired, worn-out organ to work a little harder. When you understand that herbs work either by relaxing, to allow building, or by stimulating, to allow cleansing (some herbs both stimulate for a little while and then relax), you will better appreciate the wonders of herbs.

The body must do the actual healing. Medicines possess no healing qualities; they generally can only drive the organs a little further. Herbs are foods and supply the builders of the body; they are compatible because the body was designed to use foods with which to build.

One wonder herb is a gift to modern herbalists from the Nez Percé Indian Nation—*leptotaenia*. They refer to this powerful herb as the "sacred root."

The northwestern part of the United States has a long, wet, cold winter, and, as a result, complaints caused by viruses (fever, flu, colds, etc.) are very common during the winter months. Being exposed to this difficult weather, these wonderful Indians found a natural answer to the inherent, viral-based illnesses—the sacred root—the only natural anti-viral.

This fabulous herb is found only in the mountain country where it grows on the southern slopes at an altitude of 5000 to 5500 feet above sea level. It prefers very rocky places and takes some ten to thirty years to reach maturity. It must be harvested only during a four-to-six-week period once a year.

Leptotaenia is one particular species of the thirty or so species of wild carrot which grows in the mountains. But this one specific variety is the only one which produces an effective oil.

There is, however, a caution which must be mentioned when using this herb—if you have some fungus or virus plus an alkaline system, you may have a reaction, most probably in the form of a rash. It is believed that the rash is indicative of the body's throwing off an imbedded virus if your system is alkaline. This rash is eased by soaking for about an hour in a tub of warm water into which one pound of baking soda has been dissolved. The rash occurs in only about one case in a hundred. It can be guarded against by taking about six tablespoons of vinegar in water each day for two days before using the herb.

This will help acidify the body system. It has also been determined that by combining the oil with reverse-polarity taheebo, or pau d'arco, from South America and bitter almond, that the herbs combine to form a more powerful and effective formula which doesn't produce the unwanted side effect (rash). In addition, since the taheebo is an anti-fungal and an anti-bacterial herb, the combination results in a broad spectrum formula.

If you are subject to colds and the more serious influenza, if you have a long standing infection or a low-grade infection which does not respond to other treatments, if you never feel quite "in the pink" or are suffering the "blahs" for no apparent reason, if no one can determine why you don't feel quite right, if you have at any time had a smallpox vaccination, if you suffer from hypoglycemia or diabetes, if you experience a recurring fever, or if you suffer periodic nausea and weakness every few weeks, then, perhaps the wonder herb of the Indians, leptotaenia, may be the long sought for answer for you. Chronic sore throat infections of many types, strange chills and indeterminate fevers, aches and pains of various types and various body locations, rashes and pus-filled, oozing sores, nasal catarrh, as well as many other problems respond to this miracle herb, the Nez Percé sacred root.

One doctor familiar with leptotaenia believes that it prolongs life by keeping the human system free of all viruses.

A virus has the ability to remain in the human system throughout a person's life. For this reason, some doctors have the opinion that a smallpox vaccination

given a child will show up in later life as hypoglycemia some twenty-five to thirty years after the vaccination. The virus can remain in the pancreas all the
ensuing years, damaging the beta cells. Also, many
types of cancer are known or suspected to be viral in
nature; further, many researchers hold the opinion
that these viruses live in the nerves and nerve
synapses.

The *kola nut* is included among the wonder herbs
because it is so effective and helpful to the stomach.
Many people's troubles originate in the stomach.

If the stomach doesn't function in the digestive
cycle properly, the proteins in food will be improperly processed and a Pandora's box is opened. The
food ferments in the stomach, putrifies in the colon,
and the toxic residue consisting of many toxins such
as putrescine, cadaverine, skatole, and others, seeps
into the blood stream, toxifies the liver, inundates the
kidneys, and branches out in all directions, poten-
tially causing hundreds of different disorders and dys-
functions, from sinus problems to cancer.

There are a great number of stomachics referred to
as bitters; none stands out like the kola nut.

Nothing seems to work quite as quickly as kola nut
for an upset stomach. To complete, augment, and
amplify the effectiveness of the kola nut, add goldenseal and damiana as gland stimulants, pepsin to aid
protein digestion and assimilation, pancreatin to supply the enzyme action to digest food compounds naturally, and ox bile to aid in handling fats and clean up
cholesterol in the blood and vessels.

Kelp, one of the wonder plants, is a common seaweed which contains every vital mineral needed for

sustaining bodily health. Among these minerals are: aluminum, barium, bismuth, boron, calcium, chlorine, chromium, cobalt, copper, gallium, iodine, magnesium, manganese, molybdenum, phosphorus, potassium, silicon, silver, sodium, strontium, sulfur, tin, titanium, vanadium, and zirconium.

Dulse is another form of seaweed that is finer and more pleasant tasting than kelp. Many people prefer dulse to kelp. Both varieties take all the vital mineral elements from the ocean water and convert them from inorganic substances into organic minerals, which can be used by man for health.

Living in seawater, where a treasure of minerals exists, kelp is one of the best sources of iodine, iron, potassium, and chlorine. It has a good supply of phosphorus, too. All of these minerals join to build greater brain power.

We know that seawater is a veritable treasure trove of precious minerals, so many of the plants that grow in the sea will be able to provide these same vital brain foods. Therefore, in order to have good health, one should use powdered kelp or dulse, as a flavoring agent for soups, salads, meats, baked dishes, and other dishes.

Kelp or dulse tablets taken regularly will supply the iron, phosphorus, and potassium needed by the brain and other parts of the body.

Three special brain foods are lecithin, dulse, and desiccated liver. You must have these in your diet for top-level mental powers to help you through the day. Of the three, dulse is the best if you cannot get any of the others.

It is of interest to note that maritime nations, including the Japanese, Chinese, South Sea

84

Islanders, and the Eskimos have for centuries prized seaweed among their principal vegetables. These people have been wise enough to have kelp in its varied forms as a staple in their diet. In continental Europe it is found that those living near the seashore have learned the value of seaweed, especially as a fodder for their cattle. This is particularly true in Denmark, where a dairy herd is given a supplementary feeding of dried seaweed to help increase milk production, as well as to produce richer milk.

Kelp has for many years demonstrated its value as a remedy for human ailments resulting from deficiency conditions. It has been successful in relieving glandular disturbances which often result in goiter, rickets, anemia, underweight, constipation, stomach trouble, headache, kidney disorders, eczema, neuritis, asthma, and low vitality.

Malnutrition does not come from lack of food, but from the lack of proper nutrition. Deficiency disease has reached an all-time high. In spite of the boastful claims of the authorities, we find among our own people, many of whom can purchase anything they desire to suit the palate, those who are lacking in proper foods.

Soil deficient in minerals cannot provide us with healthful foods. If we do not give our soil the proper rest and treatment so that minerals can become a part of the earth again, this world is doomed, and mankind will go down the drain by the end of this century. About the only place left for us to find good foods with minerals and herbs is the ocean floor. This has become a reservoir of accumulated wealth in chemical materials which makes the resources of the land appear as nothing in comparison.

Kelp is also used in cases of obesity, poor digestion, and obstinate constipation. It has a beneficial effect upon the reproductive organs, and a normalizing action upon the thyroid, sensory nerves, meninges, arteries, pylorus, colon, liver, gallbladder, pancreas, bile ducts, and the kidneys. Few singular plants have such a wide range of action on illnesses of the body and diseased organs.

Dulse is mild flavored, pleasant to eat, and is easy to handle. Many health authorities advise kelp or dulse for indigestion. A bottle of capsules of this valued seaweed should be kept on the medicine shelf at all times in order to relieve chronic constipation and stomach disorders and to act as an arterial cleansing agent giving tone to the walls of the blood vessels.

Dulse is helpful in cases of arterial tension due to high blood pressure and in keeping down a host of disorders.

Licorice is an herb of which there are several varieties. Its name is a corruption of the Greek words for sweet and root. It is one of the oldest and best known remedies for coughs and chest complaints. The knowledge and use of it dates back to the time of the early days of Egyptian civilization. According to some historians, the early clay tablets found on the plains of Mesopotamia (which is supposedly the birthplace of civilization) gave many uses of licorice as a medicine and as the elixir of life.

The Hindus, Greeks, Romans, Babylonians, and Chinese all knew about the value of licorice. Gopal Das, one of the ancient ECK Masters, was responsible for it being introduced into Egypt for medical purposes.

It is a perennial herb which grows in most temperate countries. It is about two to five feet high with long, dark green leaves and yellowish white or purplish flowers. The root is light brown with a sweet taste, fifty times the sweetness of cane sugar. It is a demulcent, expectorant, and laxative.

Its roots penetrate deeply into the ground and contain an abundance of valuable properties. It is a native of Greece, Asia Minor, Spain, southern Italy, Syria, Iraq, Caucasian and Transcaspian Russia, northern China, Persia, and North Africa.

Tons of licorice are used by all countries today for foods, medicines, beverages, confections, etc. The United States imports about fifty million pounds of licorice root and about half that amount of the liquid extract yearly. The root comes mainly from Iraq, Turkey, Russia, Syria, and Italy. The extract is imported mostly from Spain. Some of the licorice extract entering the United States is used by the drug industries and made into various medications because of its demulcent and expectorant properties and as a flavoring to hide the taste of other medicines. The root, made into a powder, is often used in the preparation of pills. The extract has almost replaced the powder as a remedial agent.

Much of the supply of licorice is used by the tobacco industry as a conditioning and flavoring agent and by the confectionery industry as a base for a wide variety of candies. The residual material after extraction is used as a stabilizer in the production of foam fire-extinguishers and as a fertilizer for mushrooms.

The Chinese herbalists regard licorice as a healing agent either by itself or as an ingredient in various herbal formulas. It is also used to flavor beer and ale, ice creams, and as licorice water, which is a blood purifier.

The popularity of licorice as a remedy for coughs and chest complaints goes back to the remote ages. Witch doctors, priests, healers, and physicians of the various ages of history found in the licorice root something which would alleviate man's suffering. Each utilized the hidden powers of the root of this wonder herb as a curative agent in many different types of ailments.

It has been effectively used for centuries, not only in treating conditions such as tuberculosis, coughs, hoarseness, wheezing, and shortness of breath, but it has also been found to be helpful for dropsy, constipation, fever, and as a blood purifier.

Licorice water was a popular drink in Egypt during the ancient days. The youthful Pharaoh Tutankhamen, who died in 1345 B.C., was buried with a supply of licorice root to help him on his last, long journey. It was a very popular therapeutic sweet drink for all the natives of those times. It was mostly imported from the fertile plains of Mesopotamia. It was also listed among the hundreds of drugs known during Hammurabi's reign of Babylonia.

Alexander the Great, so history says, distributed licorice root among his own troops for medical purposes, just as a modern soldier carries his own first aid supply in campaigns. The Roman legionnaires also considered licorice an indispensable ration for their grueling campaigns on the Roman frontiers. The Buddhists later adopted it as a sacred symbol for their ceremonies and rituals.

Almost anywhere one looks in man's history, licorice has been a part of the development of the culture and civilization of various nations.

Another wonder herb is *alfalfa*. Many believe that alfalfa is only fodder for animals. It is a leguminous plant, much like peas and beans; however, the leaves and sprouts are eaten rather than the seeds alone. Alfalfa was one of the first known herbs, perhaps used over two thousand years ago. The Arabs discovered its valuable properties and called it the father of all foods. It has been only recently that we have rediscovered its valuable nutritive uses.

Alfalfa is a rich source of potassium, magnesium, phosphorus, and calcium, as well as all the known vitamins — including vitamin K and niacinamide. Alfalfa is one of the richest known sources of organic salts. The depth and spread of its roots give it an opportunity to absorb the valuable nourishment from the soil.

Alfalfa is a good remedy to help balance blood pressure, for it contains all the necessary elements for softening hard arteries. Its rich iron content renders it a specific remedy for anemia, and its calcium content prevents dental problems. Many who are looking for youth and longevity would probably find it in the tea made from the dried green leaves of this wonder herb. It is sometimes called lucerne in England and South American countries, and buffalo herb in some parts of this country.

Alfalfa is believed to have originated in southwestern Asia, and historical accounts show it was first cultivated in Persia, now the country of Iran. From Persia it was taken to Greece during 500 B.C. and to

Spain in 800 A.D. The Spaniards brought it to North and South America. In 1854 alfalfa was taken to San Francisco from Chile and from there spread rapidly over the western states.

Alfalfa is rich in proteins, minerals, and vitamins. Because the root extends as deep as thirty feet into the soil, alfalfa can reach great stores of nutrients. In areas with limited rainfall, alfalfa can withstand extremes of drought.

The plant is remarkably adaptable to various climatic conditions, but it is exacting as to soil conditions and proper sowing. The effect of alfalfa on irrigated land is to increase the value per acre of subsequent crops. Alfalfa is used as a soiling crop and as pasturage. In the form of silage, alfalfa hay is fed to dairy cows, beef cattle, sheep, hogs, horses, and poultry. It is also an excellent honey crop for bees and is used to increase the vitamin content of prepared foods.

Alfalfa production in the United States averages over eighty-five million tons a year. The most important alfalfa producing states are California, Idaho, Washington, South Dakota, Kansas, and Nebraska.

It has been found that the green leaf of the alfalfa contains eight essential enzymes. They are lipase, a fat-splitting enzyme; amylase, which acts upon starches; coagulase, which coagulates milk and clots blood; emulsin, which acts upon sugars; invertase, which converts sucrose into glucose and fructose; peroxidase, which is also an oxidizing aid for the blood; pectase, an enzyme that forms a vegetable jelly substance which aids digestion; and proteases, which digest proteins.

Alfalfa serves as an aid to increase lagging appetites. There are enough minerals and enzymes in alfalfa, according to health authorities, to assist the digestion of all four classes of foods—proteins, fats, starches, and sugars.

Alfalfa as an aid for health is on the shelves of most stores in the country. Alfalfa sprouts contain the vital, cell-building amino acids and are rich in phosphorus, chlorine, silicon, aluminum, calcium, iron, magnesium, sulfur, sodium, and potassium in forms which the body can transform. It has been said that the alfalfa sprout contains over a hundred percent more protein than other grains. However, it is the chlorophyll contained in alfalfa which gives much of its healing quality for the body tissues.

The sprouts have calcium which would keep the teeth in good condition, as well as the heart and muscles. We find that alfalfa grown for human consumption is somewhat different from that which is cultivated for domestic animal use, as the fields are kept free from weeds.

Hawthorn is one of the wonder herbs used mainly in the treatment of heart diseases (as was discussed in chapter one). It is also used as a diuretic, astringent, a tonic for sore throats, dropsy, and kidney troubles.

The hawthorn is a small tree belonging to the rose family. Native to the temperate regions, it is widely cultivated for its use as an herb.

It attains a height of about thirty feet and lives to a great age. It passes a single seed-vessel to each blossom, producing a stony apple in miniature, and when ripe, is brilliant red. Throughout Europe, it is known as a very fine cardiac tonic and curative for organic and functional heart disorders. It goes by several different names — English hawthorn, may apple, mayblossom, whitethorn, haw tree, and bread and cheese tree. Its fruit, which is bright red and has a yellow pulp, remains on the tree after the leaves drop in the fall of the year.

The hawthorn was used in ancient Greece as a marriage torch. In Rome it was considered a potent charm against sorcery and witchcraft. The leaves were put in cradles of the newly born babies to bring special blessings and protection. Greek brides often used sprigs of hawthorn, and the wedding altar was adorned with its blossoms to bring a blessed future for the bride and groom.

Hawthorn has now come under serious scientific research and it is reported to be used as a base for heart medicines. A liquid extract is made from the English hawthorn which has proven to be valuable in continued therapy for certain heart troubles.

The bush, or tree, has small, serrated leaves and a profusion of tiny, white flowers which later give way to meaty red berries called haws. During World War II, the berries were discovered to have a rich vitamin C content by British government research teams, and they were given to the troops to prevent scurvy and to guard against dropsy.

Celery has the Latin name of *Apium graveolens*. The seeds are used mainly in herbal remedies. Celery is good for rheumatism, gout, and as a carminative medicine for relieving gas and colic. Celery seeds are also used as a diuretic and a tonic for improving the muscular condition of the body, as well as an aid to promote restfulness and sleep. It is cultivated in most parts of the world for domestic use.

Celery has been known for its medicinal use for several thousand years. The ancients made good use of its benefits for distraught nerves.

The stalk is rich in potassium, sodium, calcium, iron, and vitamin C. Celery is nonfattening and can be used as a nibbling food between meals for those who want to lose weight. Celery has the quality of satisfying hunger. The leaves of the celery plant contain vitamins A, B, and C, as well as potassium and sodium. The root contains potassium, sodium, calcium, iron, silicon, and vitamins A and B.

Celery is a biennial herb of the carrot family and is related to parsley. It is a native of Europe but is grown widely throughout the world. The stalks often grow twelve to thirty inches high in cultivated varieties. The stalk is greenish in color and slightly bitter to the taste. Celery seed is used as a seasoning for soups and other foods. It is also used in the pharmacy as a sedative or to disguise the flavor of drugs. In the United States, it is raised principally in California and Florida. Its production yearly is about twenty-five million crates, each weighing sixty-five pounds.

Asparagus is a member of the lily family. It was used by the Romans and Greeks in ancient times and the young shoots were considered to be good food.

The common asparagus which grows best in rich, well-drained, sandy soil, is a native of Europe and is now popular as a cultivated food in most countries of the world. The seeds are used as a substitute for coffee. In the United States, it is raised principally in California and New Jersey. It is cultivated abroad in southern Russia, Poland, and Greece to a greater extent than in other foreign countries.

The root or seed is mainly used in herbal remedies. It is said to be a treatment for various heart conditions, dropsy, gravel in the kidneys, and bladder or gallbladder ailments.

Parsley is common to our knowledge and raised nearly all over the world. It is a diuretic, carminative, tonic, aperient, and antispasmodic herb used for swollen glands, colic, dropsy, cystitis, and irritation of the kidneys and bladder.

The ancient Greeks used it two thousand years ago. Galen, one of the first physicians known in history, wrote about its benefits. During the early Roman era it was used as a sweet food for audiences at public events, like moviegoers today purchase popcorn and other things to nibble on during a picture.

Today, parsley has a place in medicine as a basic ingredient to alleviate a wide number of complaints. Many use it in Europe for various medical reasons, but mainly it is used for its properties which are essential to oxygen metabolism and maintaining the general health of the body, especially the action of the adrenal and thyroid glands. Also, it is used for vitamins A and C, which the plant contains in large amounts.

Another herb is *papaya,* a fruit of the tropical countries — especially the Americas. A native of Hawaii and the South Sea Islands, it has been brought to America where it grows well in the southern, semitropical states, and in the tropical Latin American countries.

94

It is a tree that grows twenty-five to thirty feet in height, producing a yellow melon with delicious soft inner flesh. Another species of the tree was grown in the tropics of the central Americas and its fruit was used by the Incas, Mayans, and other civilizations long before the Spaniards came to their shores.

The melon flesh is nature's finest digestant. It contains papain, a digestive enzyme which has no equal. It will digest hard foods, is active in alkaline or acid, and is of value as a neutral medium. It also assists in the digestion of other foods and is used as a digestive aid for patients who have weak stomachs.

Papaya is a source of vitamins A, B complex, C, and G, and is used in a good many types of preparations such as jams, marmalades, drinks, and fruit salads.

The powerful protein-digesting enzyme papain, which greatly resembles pepsin in its digestive action, is made into tablets and sold as an aid for protein digestion, especially for older people whose bodies have aged to the point where the stomach will not digest certain foods. It is also valuable as an active blood clotting agent to arrest bleeding. Papain is also effective in destroying intestinal worms.

We also find protein-digesting enzymes in the *pineapple*. Bromelain, similar to papain, gives valuable aid in helping to digest proteins in the stomach.

Bromelain is found in greater concentration near the skin of the pineapple and is extracted from the peelings which are a by-product of canned pineapple. Because it is so strong, people familiar with pineapple always peel the fruit, being sure to cut off all the eyes. Then, they slice the pineapple and sprinkle it lightly with salt and let it set a little while. This seems to reduce the violent action of this incredible enzyme. Bromelain is a much more violent digestant than papain and should be treated with respect. Raw pineapple can't be made into gelatin or jelly as the bromelain will digest the gelatin and stop the setting process. Canned pineapple has been processed above 170 degrees, so the bromelain action is arrested, but cooked pineapple does aid the hydrochloric acid production in the stomach, which helps digestion.

The mint family of herbs contains many useful varieties. A few members of the mint family are: calamint, cape mint, pennyroyal, peppermint, spearmint, common bugle, horehound, water mint, apple mint, hyssop, balm, bergamot mint, marjoram, sage, catnip, curled mint, horsemint, thyme, and skullcap.

When you study the characteristics of the whole family, one stands out above all the rest —*spearmint*. Spearmint regulates the delicate pH balance better than any other substance. If your body is too alkaline or too acid, spearmint will help correct it. It is helpful sometimes with oncoming allergies and sensitivities. It works on the endocrine gland system to regulate, modify, and stabilize the glandular functions. It is soothing to the nerves and supplies some very important minerals to the nerves. It is a good penetrant and will carry deep into the tissues. The oil has antibiotic qualities and pain-relieving abilities, possibly due to its ability to overcome alkalosis. It has a tendency to open capillary circulation to deep tissues, and this same action helps get circulation going in cases of sinus congestion. It is soothing to

96

the digestive system and, in mild cases, will close the cardiac valve to the stomach, thus stopping heartburn which is caused when the stomach contents pass through the valve up into the esophagus.

Another herb which has value is *peppermint*. Part of the mint family, as is spearmint, both are found throughout Europe, North Africa, and Asia Minor. These have been popular herbs since the earliest of times and have been mentioned in many of the ancient writings.

Peppermint is grown commercially in North America, Europe, and parts of Asia. Most of it in the United States is raised in the Pacific Northwest and in the Midwestern sections. It is a perennial herb, has a square stem and aromatic leaves, with aromatic oil in all its parts.

Peppermint is the best known of the mints and it is used in flavoring beverages, jellies, and sauces. It is used in herbal remedies for a wide variety of things, such as nausea, diarrhea, colic, and nervous headaches. For medicinal purposes it is classed as antispasmodic and carminative.

The whole mint family has been used in some manner or other by the magicians, priests, and physicians for thousands of years.

There are many other herbs that will be taken up in other chapters which could be classified as wonder herbs, but those we have just discussed are the better known ones and are good, all-around conditioners for man's health.

5

The Life-Giving Properties of Seeds

Those who follow the path of Eckankar, the Ancient Science of Soul Travel, are conscious of just where herbology fits into the spiritual works. It is true that those who have learned Soul Travel—that is, the movement of the inner consciousness through the lower states of life into the ecstatic states and awareness of God—can have pure freedom. But there are many within the ranks of Eckankar who are passing through the first stages of spiritual unfoldment and need some physical assistance for the body and mind.

The majority of people do not understand the laws of this physical universe and believe that they may do as they like for years, only to learn one day that a price must be paid for violating the laws of good health. Not many can live like the ancient Adepts of the mystical order in ECK known as the Order of the Vairagi.

The Adepts live in the Himalayas along the

Tibetan border. Among them, Rebazar Tarzs, the great ECK spiritual Master, is said by many to be over five hundred years old. Many of the other Adepts of this mysterious order are beyond the normal age of man.

Many of these Adepts live in the spiritual city of Agam Des. Few go to this strange place for they must visit only by invitation and then in the Atma body.

Eckankar was brought here from Venus by a little-known race which is living in Agam Des, and whom we know as the *Eshwar Khanewale,* or simply as the God-eaters. These beings are members of the Ancient Brotherhood, or Order, of the Vairagi. They attained their name, the God-eaters, from the fact that they absorb cosmic energies instead of assimilating plants and other foods.

They have an extreme longevity, like the patriarchs of the Old Testament, and in some cases even longer. However, those living in the physical body should not try to develop themselves to this extent, for herbs, medicines, and other means of handling health must be approached through the usual channels. Herbs are the aids that one obtains when he cannot be healed otherwise because of a karmic condition. The medicine, the health practitioner, and the family physician are part of maintaining good health on this plane.

So many people in desperation seek psychic and spiritual healing or go to famed spots like Lourdes to regain their health. Many are vastly disappointed and cannot understand why one person is able to come away completely cured and another does not meet with any success at all.

The whole crux of the problem is that it is a matter of survival with the individual. If a person has a good survival factor — basic personal traits such as cheerfulness, a reasonable amount of happiness in his disposition, a positive outlook on life and its problems, and keeps busy most of the time — he is likely to have good health. Even during those times when he is struck with illnesses, they are only temporary because of the nature of his disposition, which is good for his survival.

Too many persons look to spiritual healing for their health. To be frank, not everybody is able to have spiritual healing, regardless of what may be said about the many cases on record of those who have been healed. If one is high enough on the spiritual ladder there is little doubt about his receiving a healing when he makes a request. But our concern at present is for those who are unable to get any degree of health at this particular stage except through the regular channels of herbs, medicines, and chemistry.

This brings us to the point of seeds and what benefit they might afford the health seeker. It appears that for many centuries primitive man used seeds instead of meat. The reason for this was that it was easier to store seeds for the winter months when the hunters were kept in their lodges and caves by inclement weather.

These tribes also found that gathering seeds and nuts required less effort than hunting animals for food. Sometimes hunting became too dangerous and some hunters never returned. It was also discovered that some seeds had a higher protein content than meat, and while the tribesman could not figure this

101

out scientifically, he knew that there was something in the nature of seeds and nuts that made him feel just as well as when he ate meat.

Take, for example, lecithin. It is of great value to the human body for it contains a combination of fats, phosphorus, and nitrogen which forms an important part of the nerves of the brain. Most seeds provide a source of fats which do not cause cholesterol deposits. The Indians of the highlands in Central America have a high regard for the native squash and pumpkin seeds as protein, but if they were asked why, they probably could not say.

These squash grow wild in Mexico and throughout Central America. When the seeds are heated on a piece of metal over coals, they puff up like popcorn and are affectionately called *pepitas*. They are a national treat in Mexico. It is said that men who eat pepitas regularly have no signs of prostate problems.

The Japanese use sesame seeds for making meal for cooking. The Turks, Syrians, and Egyptians do the same, while in Spain and Portugal, we find that acorns, the nut of the oak tree, are cultivated for their delicacy. The Turks also use hempseed, and the Hindus and Russians eat cucumber and sunflower seeds instead of candy.

Seeds are one of God's gifts to man, for they contain all the nutrients required for health and strength in the body. Yet it has been only a few years since we believed that seeds were something other than food for animals and birds.

Sprouted seeds are a valued raw food which we have been neglecting all these years. They have an exceptional richness in vitamins, including plant hormones which stimulate the endocrine glands. We find that the Asians, especially the Chinese and Hindus, are great users of sprouted seeds.

Sprouts are important because they are easily digested and contain a more complete protein than the seeds they were sprouted from. When the seeds sprout, their proteins are changed and a broader spectrum of amino acids is produced. The vitamin content is increased dramatically, some of the minerals become more assimilable, and the enzymes increase geometrically.

The sulfur-bearing proteins of sprouts are strengthened so they do not break down as quickly. Sprouted beans can be cooked and tenderized at a low temperature (180–190 degrees) in just 45 minutes, and this way will not produce the large quantity of bowel gas. The sulfur in beans is important to the health of the individual because the sulfur is bonded to an amino acid, which is helpful in producing hormones and glandular substances. The sulfur also acts as a tissue detoxifier to strip the toxins out of the body.

Sprouting is not difficult. Anyone, even small children, can be taught to sprout seeds. The sprouts can be used in salads, on sandwiches, added to drinks in the blender or to soup just before serving.

Directions: 1) Find a clean canning jar (the size will depend on the quantity of seeds you wish to sprout) and a piece of plastic screen (window screen)—a strip three inches long will make a number of closures. 2) Place two tablespoons of small seeds or four tablespoons of the larger seeds in the jar. It is better to sprout small amounts that can be started every two or three day; this will provide a continuous supply of fresh sprouts. 3) Cut the screen so that it is about a half inch larger than the ring on the lid, place it over the top of the jar, and screw the ring on the jar with only the screen covering the opening. 4) Leaving the screen in place, pour a cup of fresh water in the jar with the seeds. A few drops of Chlorox or a magnet taped to the side of the jar is said to reduce the growth of bacteria. Let the seeds soak for a few hours or overnight. 5) Pour off the water and lay the jar on its side so that air can reach the seeds. The jar should be kept in the dark and at room temperature. 6) Without removing the screen, rinse the sprouts with fresh water at least two times a day. Each time, drain off the water and lay the jar on its side. 7) Harvest in about three to six days, depending on the seeds used.

Most any seeds can be used to sprout. The smaller seeds such as clover, alfalfa, radish, or cabbage will produce nice sprouts, as will mung beans, peas, sunflower seeds, or squash seeds. These are only general instructions; you may wish to experiment or study different approaches to sprouting.

When cooking beans of all kinds, you can include some of the sprouting steps to increase the nutritional value of the beans. *Directions:* 1) Soak the beans overnight in a pan of water. 2) Next day pour off the water and save it in the refrigerator. 3) Place the beans in a wide, low pan about three to four deep and cover with a damp towel. 4) Sprout the beans for two nights and a day, rinsing the beans twice a day. Do not sprout for longer than this, as the flavor will be changed. 5) Boil the water you originally soaked the beans in for five minutes. 6) Turn down the heat and add the sprouted beans. Cook at 180 degrees, just under boiling, for forty-five minutes or until a bean, pressed between thumb and finger, forms a firm paste. Use in any recipe calling for cooked beans. Generally, if soybeans are used, the sprouts are removed and used separately.

At the present time, there are hundreds of farms in this country that are devoted entirely to seed production for human consumption. Before this relatively recent interest in the nutritional value of seeds, farmers kept their seeds, like the pumpkin and others, in order to replant and grow another crop. All they were interested in was the flesh of the pumpkin to feed families. Yet today we find seed farms practically everywhere and seed companies that specialize in this particular market. It is interesting how the seed market has developed over the years.

Live seeds and grain have been found in Egyptian burial tombs several thousand years old. Seeds, with their durable covering, their insulated protection, may be preserved for a greater length of time than most herbs and plants.

Seeds, especially those of the cereal plants, form the greater part of the food for mankind. As early farmers spread north, south, east, and west from their native lands to countries where they found better lands for crops, new ideas were developed. Rye grew at low levels in Asia, but had a better yield in the uplands. In the same manner, oats and rye displaced wheat in northern Europe. Meanwhile, different millets were grown in Abyssinia and in northern China, where rice was developed. The latter spread southward and finally became part of the cultivated crops of the valley of the Ganges, the Southeast Asian countries, and southern China.

Pungent and aromatic seeds have been used for many purposes in the past as well as in the present. Coriander seeds were used by the Israelites at the feast of the Passover. They were also highly esteemed by Hindus, Arabs, and Egyptians. Caraway seeds have been used for centuries as a flavoring in cookery, to add relish to baked fruits, breads, and cakes. Fenugreek seeds are used as a condiment in Egypt and for curries in India. The natives of India also use fenugreek seed for making a gruel with sugar and milk. Fenugreek, when used as a tea or in powdered form, becomes an excellent blood cleanser.

In the Middle Ages, *hempseed* was used as a charm, but today it is put to better use as birdseed; its oil is used in the manufacture of soaps.

Fennel seeds were used by the Romans to make the taste of medicines more pleasant. Today the seed is used in stock for soups and other cooking, as well as to flavor absinthe and liqueurs.

Mustard is a seed known for its nutritional value since the early days of man. It is a pungent herb of the pepper order, and plants are cultivated for their seed. There are several types of mustard plant, but the commercial mustard which we find on the kitchen shelf for cookery is the black mustard plant and the white mustard plant. The seeds are ground and mixed for table mustard. Powdered mustard is also used as a medicinal substance. Powdered mustard seed is sometimes given by physicians as a powerful emetic. The mustard seed is often used for its rubefacient and counterirritant effect in the form of plasters.

Anise is valued as a carminative, antispasmodic, and pectoral. It is a plant which has an erect stem, branching from twelve to eighteen inches high, pithy, striated, and angular. Its petals are white. It was originally a native of Egypt, Syria, and the nearby islands of the eastern Mediterranean Sea. However, it has become a domestic plant and has been raised abundantly on farms and in gardens throughout the world.

Anise is used for flavoring candies and medicine. It forms one of the bases for common cough drops sold commercially. It is a little seed with much flavor which has been used as a basic ingredient from ancient times, as has the oil, which is distilled from the anise fruit. Anise has many medicinal uses, one of which is to treat a dry, hacking cough in bronchitis and asthma. It is used as a flavoring in curry powder, cheese, cookies, sweet pickles, and liqueurs. Its oil, besides being used for masking the taste of unpleasant medicines and to perfume toilet articles, makes a useful ointment against lice and insects. Also, the oil is often used as a lure for fish bait and trapping small animals.

Senna is often used for medicinal purposes as a cathartic and cholagogue. It is a small shrub found to have originated in Egypt, Nubia, and Arabia. The early Arab and Greek physicians were among the first to use the leaves and pods of this plant as medicine. Most of the senna used commercially is from Egypt and Ethiopia. American senna is weaker and is usually combined with aromatics.

Wild carrot seeds are used for colic, dropsy, and kidney stones.

Annatto is a bush which grows in the tropical areas of the Americas. Its seeds are used to color butter, cheese, soups, rice, cosmetics, pomades, soaps, silks, and varnishes.

The *betel nut* is widely known as a seed which the natives of Southeast Asia chew. Mixed with honey, syrup, or butter, betel nuts are used in veterinary medicine as a vermifuge.

Cardamom is a member of the ginger family, native to the Oriental countries. Its seeds are used for curry powders, flavoring foods, incense, and perfumes. The seeds are helpful to ease indigestion and flatulence.

Pumpkin seeds have a good many uses. In China these seeds are a symbol of health. It is believed that they are valuable for medicinal purposes. It is said they have a vitalizing effect on the prostate glands. Pumpkin seeds contain an abundance of the B vitamins, with smaller amounts of vitamin A, as well as calcium and protein.

Fennel seeds are used for flavoring soups and boiled fish. The ancients believed that by eating fennel and using its seeds for flavoring, they gained strength, courage, and longevity. Now fennel is used mainly as a carminative and stomachic, for stomachache in infants, and similar complaints.

Cumin seed is mentioned in the ancient sacred writings and by the early Greek authors. It was a popular household medicine and was also used as a spice during the Middle Ages. Cumin is still used as a condiment to flavor foods such as bread, soup, rice, pickles, cheese, curry powders. It is an aid for digestion, helps with colic and some types of headaches.

Fenugreek seed was popular with the old Mediterranean civilizations. The seed contains niacin, phosphorus, lecithin, and iron. It is sometimes used as a substitute for codfish oil in treatment of rickets and anemia. Fenugreek is an excellent blood cleanser and is effective when brewed as a tea for relief of sore throats. It is also used as a food for horses and cattle.

Flax seeds are also useful, having numerous medicinal and economic uses. Flax is used in the base preparations for cough medicines, digestive problems, catarrh, and in inflammation of lungs, intestines, and urinary passages.

Guarana is an herb which comes from the Amazon jungles. The Amazon Indians pound the seeds into meal. A tea can also be made from the seeds. It is good for furnishing protein and keeping up strength of the body. Since guarana is high in caffeine, it should be used sparingly and with care.

Psyllium seed is a common weed in southern Europe. It has been used for centuries as a laxative and sometimes for poultices.

The *parsnip* plant has a seed which is a good diuretic. Be careful in harvesting parsnip as some species, such as the water parsnip, are very poisonous.

Sumac berries, when beaten into a powder, stop hemorrhages and are used as a diuretic. Since there are species of sumac that are poisonous, special care should be taken for proper identification.

The *sesame* plant is an annual herb, with pale or rose-colored flowers, that grows to a height of three feet. It is a native of India, grown for its seeds, which are eaten as food. The seeds are also ground into a nut butter which is spread on bread, rolls, biscuits, and cookies. The seeds yield an oil used in cooking, for lighting, and lubrication. The pale yellow, emollient oil is also used to anoint the body and hair in some religious ceremonies. This oil is sometimes known as gingelly oil. In India, sesame seeds are often used for the treatment of piles, constipation, and other intestinal troubles.

The seeds of the sesame plant have always been favored by the ECK Masters as a rich source of vitamins, minerals, and protein. Sesame seeds contain an abundance of calcium and lecithin. The use of sesame in this country was developed and promoted by the natural food industry. Sesame has become a household staple and is a valuable aid to the human diet. It is used extensively in cooking, in the manufacture of margarine, and in commercial products such as salad oils and cosmetics. The sesame seed is now domesticated and grows in all parts of the tropical world. There are processing plants in Ecuador, Mexico, Peru, Nicaragua, and Costa Rica.

Sesame oil is not odorous, has a sweet taste, and will keep for long periods without becoming rancid, if it is stored properly. Containing a natural antioxidant, sesame oil will keep longer than other oils. But if exposed to light or heat, it will become rancid like any other oil, so it should be stored in a cool, dark place. Because sesame oil has a low smoke point (the temperature at which the oil breaks down and smoky fumes are given off), it is important to keep the cooking temperatures low. After being heated, sesame oil will become rancid. Peanut oil, with a much higher smoke point, is often a better choice for cooking because it is safer and will not become rancid as quickly after heating.

A note about oils in general: When cooking oils of any type are heated, they begin to break down, becoming rancid and forming compounds which can be carcinogenic. This process cannot be reversed. There are businesses that will recycle and hydrogenate the oil used in restaurants, which improves the taste and smell but does not remove the rancid compounds. Consider this factor when eating fried foods at a restaurant.

When purchasing cooking oils, look for expeller-expressed oils rather than cold-pressed or chemically-treated oils. Buy your oil in small containers, store them in a cold, dark place, and try to use the oil within two to three weeks. Freshness is very important.

Along with milk, meat, eggs, cheese, and nuts, we find that seeds are a good source of protein. For example, sesame seeds are similar to almonds in their composition, being an excellent protein food, containing methionine, which is effective for liver complaints.

Sunflower seeds are rapidly becoming one of the staples in the diets of America. They have been the staple food in the Balkan countries for many years, and since we have adopted the sunflower seed for eating purposes, it appears that general health has improved. The seed is extremely rich in methionine, and provides more amino acids than liver.

The Greeks and ancient Romans were great enthusiasts for sunflower seeds. When the early French explorers made trips along the shores of the Great Lakes, they found the Indian tribes cultivating the sunflower for its seeds. When the Spaniards came to the shores of tropical America, they found the natives in Peru and Mexico harvesting the sunflower. The sunflower is grown in Russia today and its seeds are used as food. Oil cakes are made from the sunflower seed and used as fodder for cattle and horses during the cold Russian winter when food is scarce.

Sunflower seeds contain valuable nutritional elements. Its oil is excellent for use in salads and cooking. Research shows that the seed oil is an excellent aid in reducing the cholesterol level in the blood. The seeds contain an abundance of vitamins and minerals, are rich in B-complex vitamins, and supply an excellent source of protein. They also contain vitamin A and a high content of phosphorus and calcium. The oil is used as an herbal remedy for bronchitis and as an aid for healthy eyes.

Seeds are valuable nutritionally and can be eaten as healthy snacks in place of sweets or processed-food items. Processed sugar robs the body of vitamin B which is so important to good health. Thiamine, or B_1, is said to be the portion destroyed. Thiamine is the element that aids the metabolism of carbohydrates, including the sugars and starches. Sugars and starches, eaten in their natural form, do not have the same effect on the body, for the thiamine can readily metabolize the sugar or starch present in natural food. Sugar of all kinds not only robs the body of vitamin B_1, B_2, and vitamin C, but also reduces the amount of hydrochloric acid in the stomach. The sugars and starches are changed into glycogen, and

112

this is in turn converted to glucose — a source of energy for the body — by use of the B vitamins, which are thus depleted. Corn syrup and fructose from corn syrup are the worst offenders in depleting the B vitamins because they are processed so quickly. Because corn syrup is a less expensive source of sweetening than cane or beet sugar, it is used in almost every processed food. Read the labels.

Many historical characters have been greatly addicted to sweets — Hitler, Napoleon, Queen Elizabeth I, Alexander the Great, Stalin, Julius Caesar, and Queen Victoria, to name a few. It does seem likely that the rulers named subjected themselves to the metabolic paradox of creating a condition of low blood sugar by eating too much sugar.

If the diet is balanced, then we should have little worry about the problem of good health. Sugar is necessary, but not at the expense of other needs of the body. An excess of sugar in the blood stimulates the pancreas to produce so much insulin that not only is the excess sugar removed from the bloodstream, but practically all the blood glucose as well. Insufficient glucose is left in the blood for the demands of the brain cells. As a result, suspicion, depression, inability to think clearly, and anger become the effects in the individual whose intake of sweets is too high. He becomes somewhat indifferent, and he reaches a state in which he becomes cruel to others, sadistic in manner and thought, and his deeds are often marked by outstanding errors of judgment.

The most famous vegetarian of our times was Adolf Hitler. In order to compensate for the lack of zest in his diet, which was likely due to lack of meat protein, he went to extremes with sweets. This seems to be a somewhat common problem with vegetarians generally. A visit to any vegetarian restaurant will show all sorts of sweets, cakes, and pastries on the menu. Of course, many of these rich foods are made from whole grains, natural sugars, and such, but at the same time, many of them are not. Some who can be called "amateur vegetarians" ruin their health by trying to eat in this manner, and they learn sooner or later that a strict regimen does not work for their health. The races of people who have had to be vegetarians have been more warlike and have had more problems internally than those who maintained balanced nutrition within their respective countries.

It appears that there is a substance in the stomach which is required if one is to be a vegetarian. This substance aids in the digestion of the long molecules of vegetable protein into amino acids that can be used by the body. Without proper digestion of the vegetable proteins, toxins form which are absorbed into the bloodstream and affect the entire body.

For the body to produce this digestive substance, one must be born of parents who have lived on a vegetarian diet, or one should have had very little meat before the age of eight. If a mature person begins a restricted vegetarian diet and does not have this digestive substance in his system, he may feel fine for a while. But after a period of time, he may start to feel worn out, listless, or tired all the time. Health problems may begin to appear. As little as one cubic inch of fish twice a week could benefit this type of person.

It is not that one way of eating is better than another, but that each of us must find what is best for his own particular needs.

It appears that those persons who are reared in a home where the conditions do not warrant too many sweets, including candies and sugarized soft drinks, have a greater chance of being happier, with an opportunity for longevity.

Perhaps the cause of the rise of crime today could be traced to this particular lack of good nutrition. At least some of it might, for many people apparently want only what the pleasure principle within them demands, and this is certainly true in the line of nutrition. If left alone, most of these people would take alcohol, sugared drinks, candies, pies, pastries, and cakes as their main food element.

It is noted that Denmark, which has a high suicide rate, has an average yearly intake of 124 pounds of sugar per person. What does this mean? Are the people having problems due to an excess of sweets in their diets? It is a matter to be considered. The United States has an intake per person per annum of some one hundred pounds. This is dropping slightly each year. Less candy has been sold each year for the past ten years, the sugar beet industry is in hard times, and the sugar cane industry of Hawaii is suffering financially.

Most people do not need this much sugar and starch. They would get sufficient carbohydrates if their diet consisted of raw and cooked vegetables, fish, and chicken. If they are underweight, they could have a high-carbohydrate meal in the evening.

If you have a craving for sugar and have a difficult time controlling it, perhaps your B vitamins are depleted. A good B complex vitamin taken for a couple of weeks will often cause the craving for sweets to disappear. A craving for sweets may also reflect a serious protein deficiency. Balanced protein is required, and one should not combine carbohydrates with proteins. Shrimp is an excellent source of protein. If you need extra energy, two or three raw egg yolks (fertile if possible) blended into twelve ounces of dark grape juice once or twice daily will quickly build up your protein balance.

It is said that artificial sweeteners have the same effect upon the blood in the body as refined sugar. If this is at all true, then anyone with a sweet tooth had best learn to discipline this habit, rather than succumbing to the problems it might bring. In any case, one would be far better off eating fruits which are freshly picked than pies, desserts, and other sweets.

The vegetarian who is motivated by a religious creed takes his stand on the moral issue that eating flesh is against the principles of spirituality. Anyone who is a chela of Eckankar knows that after he has become proficient in Soul Travel and can go into the Fifth, Soul, Plane, there is no moral right or wrong, only complete responsibility for every act — no beauty and no ugliness, only the one reality. Those who believe that vegetarianism is an asset to their spiritual growth are mistaken about the moral issue. However, there is agreement that one might feel better if he were a very light eater of animal flesh, substituting fish for beef, avoiding pork and lamb, and using chicken occasionally. Turkey could be reserved for festive times, a few times a year.

If one is going to follow the path of the vegetarian, he had best examine his own physical makeup and learn if he is able to do so. It is the same in regard to

116

fasting. Not everybody can fast, for it is not within the chemical makeup of their physical being to do so. Those who can, usually are sensible about the matter and attempt it a little at a time in order to harden their bodies so they can get used to whatever suffering they might encounter at the beginning of the fast. They usually fast a few days in the beginning, then wait a few days or weeks before going longer. In this manner they work up the strength and psychological preparation which must always go with a fast of any duration.

Fasting is as old as the human race. When nature did not provide a fast by droughts or floods, a religious fast was likely to take place.

The first things we must learn are the laws of biology, which are actually the fundamental principles of the nature of Kal, the negative force. Man is subject to the trials and processes of evolutionary spiritual growth in his struggle for existence and survival. If we seem to escape trials, it is because the group to which we belong has protected us, or because we, as chelas of Eckankar, have been surrounded by the Living ECK Master's love, which wards off certain trials. He will take care of all his chelas up to a point, allowing them the lesson of some experience, which is unique to each individual, to undo some karma.

The first thing that man learns is that life is competitive. When food is plentiful, life is peaceful; when food becomes scarce and man looks for anything to eat, life is violent. Animals eat one another without qualm; civilized men consume one another by due process of law. When men cooperate, there is an increase of social development, but this, too, is a

117

tool and a form of competition. War is a nation's way of eating; it is the ultimate form of competition.

Man will eat in some form or another—whether it is the devouring of something to satisfy a hunger, or being a member of a group that declares war on another. As long as man is in the physical body and living in the human state of consciousness, he is in competition with others and must do something to survive.

This is why fasting should be done voluntarily, with the idea in mind that it is for spiritual growth and bodily health. If anyone fasts for any other reason, such as to force someone or some group into accepting his ideas or making changes, he has only made karma for himself. This is poor karma, indeed, for he must live through other lives in order to overcome that which he has forced another to do. Force in any form will not work, whether it be by fasting to change others, or by employing weapons, propaganda, and the force of ideas.

Fasting in ancient times was necessary for some religions. It appears that this was a part of the spiritual growth of people who were seeking God. To tell anyone today to fast for any length of time would be like taking their property away; few, if any, could abstain from food of any nature for one day. But again, this depends upon the individual's psychological makeup and his physical endurance. There have been studies made of fasting in health circles and varied systems and ideas have been developed.

The complete or partial fast will free the body from any physical blockage that might be bothering it. When food is withheld the body starts feeding on

118

itself from within. The inner healer takes over, and what is least essential to the body is used or released in some manner.

The first two or three days of the fast are the hardest. After that, most hunger pangs disappear and the individual seems to be free of any disagreeable feelings in the stomach and body. If one is not used to fasting, he should try only two or three days at first, and he should have the advice of the family physician or health authority before attempting it. If he should later feel that his endurance can manage a longer fast, then he can try whatever seems possible. However, he should not attempt the thirty day fast, which was part of the development of the spiritual giants. There is too much misery in starting a fast of this nature and too much disappointment if one has to stop within a few days after starting.

Two important points regarding fasting. First, if you are a confirmed faster and have been on several extended fasts, be sure to instruct the subconscious mind that you want your body to be well and that you are not starving it but wish to make it healthy. It is possible for the subconscious to believe that you wish to be rid of the body, and it will try to assist with a tendency toward accidents to fulfill this supposed wish.

Second, a long fast of twelve or more days may endanger your health, as the radioactive elements and lead that is stored in the liver will be released into the bloodstream. Generally this happens around the eighteenth day, but could happen earlier or later depending upon the individual. When these elements come out of the liver, they may settle in the bones where they can cause cancer.

119

In former times, people did not have this problem, but we are in the age of the atom and are confronted with radiation all around us. A short fast of one to five days, repeated often, seems to do no harm.

The initiates of Eckankar, of the Second Circle and above, are requested to abstain from food each Friday. If unable to do this, they are given permission to take a partial fast, or one with fruit juices only. In cases of the elderly, or those who are unable to do this, it is requested that they have a mental fast for this day; that is, to keep all thinking and action of a positive nature.

6

Herbs and Karmic Conditions
of Man

Many fashions are forming different faces for society. None of these are "revolutions," as the journalists tag them, but merely fads, which crop up from time to time in any social order.

The only real revolution is the enlightenment of the mind and unfoldment of Soul for spiritual growth, and the only real emancipation is as Soul. Therefore, the only real revolutionists are the Adepts of the Ancient Order of Vairagi, the Masters of Eckankar. They are the ones who have had a secret influence on world history since the beginning of time. They are the ones who have gradually guided men through the ages, teaching them how to have social relationships with one another and how to promote the universal good for the benefit of all civilizations.

Within this overall pattern of life, there has been the gradual discovery of herbs and their beneficial effect upon the human body. Man could not be given knowledge of all things at the beginning of his time on earth. If he had had this knowledge, there would have been little purpose for his being here. Man constantly looks outward to find the answers to life's problems. He fails to look inward, to the subjective, the inner life, the center where the SUGMAD dwells, or God, as IT is known to the material world.

The lower planes are the Physical, Astral, Causal, and Mental (includes the subconscious, or Etheric Plane). The Soul Plane, which is the fifth, is the dividing line between the lower planes and the higher worlds. These lower planes were established for the education of Soul as to Its divine origin. After many incarnations and participation in all problems of life, including the gathering of karma, both good and bad, the resolution of much of it and the retaining of some of it, Soul comes to the stage of Its spiritual unfoldment where It meets the Living ECK Master, who assists It in gaining Self-Realization, the reason for Its being here on earth. When an individual receives the initiation from the Master, then all karmic conditions start resolving, and Soul will not have to return to this world again for rebirths. It has finished with the Wheel of the Eighty-Four, the circle of deaths and rebirths.

What has this got to do with herbs? We must think about the type of body that one individual has in comparison with another individual, and about keeping the varied types of bodies well. One learns to develop his own positivity, usefulness, and balance. He can gain control of himself when he learns whether his body is influenced by oxygen, nitrogen, hydrogen, carbon, manganese, magnesium, potassium, sodium, calcium, silicon, phosphorus, or a combination of any of these, such as calcium, carbon, and sulfur. These minerals are found in herbs and plants. When one learns how to preserve the minerals in vegetables and meats, then he can begin to build and maintain good health. But we must also think very carefully about the karmic conditions of man and their relationship to herbs.

In the beginning, I want to point out that zodiacal signs play an important part in the karmic conditions of every individual. A wandering Soul making Its way from birth to birth may be required to pass through each of the signs of the zodiac, spending a certain number of lives in each, working off the karma which must be collected and resolved within every sign of the zodiacal wheel. This is called the Wheel of the Eighty-Four for the number of lacs one spends going through the signs of the zodiac.

One spends so many lacs in each sign. A lac is equivalent to 100,000 years. Each Soul will spend at least eighty-four lacs going around the zodiacal circle, an average of seven lacs in each sign. He must work out the karmic conditions which come with each sign. Therefore, he would spend at least 8,400,000 lives in this universe before Soul would be purified — that is, perfected so that It can go on into the heavenly worlds.

Man has one way of breaking from the Wheel of the Eighty-Four. That is finding the Mahanta, the Living ECK Master, who will train him and eventually initiate him into the mysteries of Eckankar. When one has been initiated, most of his karma will be broken and run off in this lifetime. He will have a straight path into the heavenly world and will never have to return to this material universe again.

Now we must think in terms of which herbs and plants are best for one who has karmic conditions to run off. The various types of persons must be brought into focus through their traits and the minerals each type requires, which correlate with the signs of the zodiac.

Oxygen people are those who are chemically adapted to the plants and herbs which have much oxygen in their nature. These people generally have qualities of aggressiveness, practicality, positivity, and a great deal of confidence in themselves. They are usually dark-skinned, dark-eyed, broad-faced, solid, and muscular. These people use a great deal of oxygen because of their physical and mental energies which require extra work for the heart, muscles, tissues, and cells.

Those who are of this oxygen nature have a karma which, with too much indulgence in foods, especially rich diets, results in overweight, heart ailments, aggressiveness, vanity, attachment to material things, imperfect blood, and kidney problems.

The minerals calcium, potassium, phosphorus, and sulfur, are ones which are very beneficial for oxygen people. The legume family (peas, beans, and clovers) is able to extract this group of minerals from the earth. The legumes have nitrogen-fixing bacteria which inhabit nodules on the roots of these plants. These bacteria have the ability to convert nitrogen in the atmosphere into a form which plants can use to form proteins. Otherwise, the nitrogen in the air is inert and not usable by plants.

124

The bacteria also enrich the soil with nitrogen in the form of nitrates and nitrites, two oxygen carriers. Nitrates contain three atoms of oxygen for each atom of nitrogen, while nitrites contain two atoms of oxygen for each of nitrogen. By forming nitrogen compounds which include potassium and sodium, the nodules help the plants take in these needed minerals.

This brings us to the next type of person, the *nitrogen type*. This type has a tendency to be pessimistic. These people even appear pessimistic, for they are heavy, stocky, dark in coloring, and usually wear frowns. Unfortunately, they consume too much nitrogen in the foods they eat, and this dilutes their oxygen. This tends to decrease the oxygen activity in the body, making them inactive and giving them the look of laziness.

They have karmic problems with the digestive tract and with elimination; they tend to be overweight, slow in thought and motion, and to suffer feelings of oppression when living in the city or in crowded areas.

Because all proteins contain nitrogen and nitrogen suppresses oxygen, consuming large quantities of heavy, animal protein will take away more oxygen, suppressing activity. This is why this type of person must be very careful about having a balanced diet. For this reason it can be said again that, when we begin to break down categories of people, one person can be a vegetarian and another cannot. It is now that one can begin to see why he might have an affinity for one kind of food over another.

We are not only dealing with individual types, but also with national and racial groups, according to their characteristics, habits, and culture. History will bear this out.

Next is the *hydrogen type*. When hydrogen is missing in the body, the individual has flabby muscles and tissues. Combined with oxygen and nitrogen, hydrogen is one of the elements needed by the body to keep the muscles taut and in tone. Those who are of the hydrogen type are usually strong, muscular people who enjoy physical work and a great deal of exercise. They seldom tire, because they take their work or exercise passively and conserve their energies. This gives them the appearance of having great endurance and the ability to work long periods without resting. They are rotund, blue-eyed, brown-haired, and large-headed.

The karmic pattern of life here includes the chance of losing a certain amount of vital energy, which could result in muscular tremors later in life. The hydrogen types are apt to have congestion of the lower intestines and bowels. There is also a tendency toward dropsy, heart weakness, and some respiratory troubles. The diet should be watched very carefully and kept more to the light, dry type of foods.

The next type is the *carbon category*. These people are usually fleshy in body and spend most of their time trying to get out of work. Because they are indisposed to work, they become inactive and retiring, lacking fire because they have upset the chemical balance of their bodies by too many sweets and starches. This type is usually overweight and babyish looking.

If the individual cannot burn off the carbon in the body properly, he feels weak most of the time. The

126

greater the consumption of carbon, the greater the need for oxygen. A small amount of oxygen and a great amount of carbon will result in a small burnoff of the latter and results in weak and flabby muscles. The carbon people have poor bones, for carbon has a poor affinity for oxygen. They crave sugar (which contains carbon) for energy and heat, but they do not have enough oxygen intake to burn the carbon properly and produce muscle energy. Unless there is proper diet and sufficient exercise, they become lethargic and weak. Many carbon people have weak backs and spines, due to a lack of iron, poor digestive systems, and poor bones.

The *manganese type* generally have good minds, often very brilliant. They are slender with thin faces and prominent jaws. Their coloring is usually blondish or neutral, which gives them an old appearance. Manganese is needed in the body to overcome laziness, sterility, and marital weakness. It is also needed for nerve health, solid bone structure, good digestion, and general overall body utilization, as well as to build resistance against illness.

The manganese people are generally impatient, uncertain, disturbed by noise and clamor. They are highly nervous and prone to many errors and some accidents. They are apt to worry about even the most minute details. Sometimes they are unable to control their emotions, bursting into weeping or excessive laughter, even giggling, and sometimes a few will use violent language, which is shocking to themselves. They seem to lack control within themselves, giving way to things, then in reflection, wondering

127

what happened. These are karmic conditions which can be corrected by diet.

If manganese becomes balanced in their bodies, they will be likely to improve their attitudes, their outlook on life, and have a far happier disposition. Their diet should consist of neutral foods such as pecans, olive oil, coconut, and eggs — plus the manganese foods, which are blueberries, lettuce, pineapple, wheat and bran cereals.

The *magnesium type* is highly restless, muscular, somewhat heavy, with dark brown hair and a flexible body, even to the extent of being "double-jointed." The magnesium people need a good vegetable, fruit, and nut diet, which should be offset by seafoods and lean beef. They need both magnesium and calcium in their diet. Occasionally, those of this type are not at all interested in close relations with others, which is a state of emotional instability sometimes seen.

This is part of the karmic pattern which one must go through if he is this type of person. However, this karma is not entirely without some sort of resolution, provided he places himself under his family physician or the proper health authorities, who have knowledge of the various categories of persons. Of course, there is always the chance that one will try to analyze himself according to these different types. This would be a mistake, for few people have the insight to look into themselves and see what is wrong. They need the experts to do this, and if at all possible, they should go to a reliable health counselor and not call upon every psychic or fortune-teller in the telephone book. Although psychics may have the ability to say

128

what is wrong, they do not have the spiritual authority to pronounce their findings.

The *potassium person* is one who has greater recuperative powers than the others. However, if he has reached a low ebb of vitality and energy, he is liable to have periods of instability. These people are usually small or of medium height. They live better in domestic peacefulness, because they are naturally of a timid nature and are very serious.

If there is a lack of potassium balance in the body, this type of individual will suffer from pyorrhea and eye troubles. The potassium people usually have red or light brown hair, affable dispositions, and full faces. They have an affectionate nature and a constant wish for family life.

The karmic pattern here is one of hypertension, which may affect the heart, throat, nose, and sinuses. A person in this category generally has a cough which has been with him since childhood. His body is usually very thin with nerve weakness. Often his mind is in poor condition with no strong memory and an inability to handle complex details. These people usually are vegetarians or near-vegetarians. They get their potassium and calcium from fruit.

Often, if one is of this chemical nature, he will be extremely nervous and a great worrier. He will be moving about at night when others wish to sleep. This takes away his normal rest and makes him very susceptible to certain health problems.

The *sodium group* of people are more or less manual laborers. If not, they enjoy sports and other outdoor activities. They are usually hard workers and have stocky, muscular bodies.

Sodium acts upon the blood, secretions in the body, the membranes of the vital organs, including the throat and the alimentary canal. If there is not enough sodium in the body, the stomach walls will weaken and acidity will result, causing the person to lash out with a verbal storm and become extremely sarcastic. The lack of sodium also causes mental depression.

Besides these points, there is a pattern of gall-stones, throat trouble, bladder problems, slow elimination, slow recovery after an illness, and a tendency to overeat, which comes from not having the proper diet.

The *calcium type* is usually slender with a large skeletal structure. He has a thin face, deep eyes, and his hair is usually brown. He is slow moving in his actions, but he works hard at anything he must do. His expression is always intent and serious, but he is tenacious in nature, and he will finish a job regardless of the cost to himself or to his health.

He is stiff in his disposition, as well as in his body and limbs, because this is the nature of the calcium type. He will normally have longevity in life, but he should always be temperate in everything, including physical and mental labor. He is pretty good at a vegetarian diet, but he must have physical and emotional warmth in his life. He has trouble with his elimination because of his eating habits, and he should pay attention to a laxative diet consisting of foods that would help him in this area daily.

These foods include whole foods, grains, cereals, fruits, and vegetables, those which have soluble fiber and are high in calcium. Alkalizers such as strawberries, dates, figs, prunes, grapes, oats, bran of all kinds, and fresh vegetables are also beneficial. Do not use head lettuce or oak leaf lettuce as both of these contain an opium-type compound called lactucarium, and it paralyzes the bowels and contributes to constipation. Refined cereals, white flour products, meats, and the high potassium foods, which are acidifiers, can also promote constipation.

Because the calcium person's disposition is generally serious and seldom changes, he can be expected to be gruff and direct in dealing with people. This is part of his karma and must be expected of him. Unless one knows this, the calcium type can certainly upset one. It is most important that people understand one another — i.e., their chemical types — before entering into marriage. If more people did this, there would be fewer separations and divorces in this world.

Too many people expect love to resolve their problems. Love is not the ultimate answer to the human element here in this physical world, but understanding is. Once we begin to understand and let compassion guide us, we are no longer in the hands of the Kal (the negative) forces.

Many do not understand that this negative force is very subtle, and it takes many turns and diverse means to keep us in its hands. Perhaps Socrates struck the keynote for defeating this negative force within ourselves by stating, "Know thyself." This is Truth, but we are so wrapped up in the astral and materialistic forces which are the basis of the negative that it is seldom that we can attain Truth anywhere.

The *silicon people* are overactive people, for they must hurry and rush about doing all sorts of things, some perfectly useless and others for good reasons. They are people with a certain amount of nimbleness, and they are constantly happy about all life.

Many of them are constant talkers, often boastful. They are quite wide-eyed, their hair is dark, sandy, or light brown. The silicon people are good party-goers, for they are open and friendly; but their energies drive them so much that they seldom are good thinkers. Their most prominent feature is that their ears stand out from the head. They cannot do heavy work, and if they do, will generally collapse from exhaustion.

Their karmic pattern is that their skin is very susceptible to the elements. They should rest often, because of a lack of energy, and most of all, they should take a rest from talking. They need natural sugars and salts. Silicon is found in onions, spinach, parsnips, pumpkins, strawberries, asparagus, celery, and lettuce. Silicon helps with the disposition. If the silicon type will take care of their skin, which can develop a malignancy, there is a good chance of these individuals living to a ripe old age.

The *phosphorus type* of person has a pear-shaped head when looked at from any angle. There is a mental alertness in the faces of the phosphorus people which shows a desire for reading, studying, and learning. Their hair is brown, and their eyes are usually blue or gray. The neck is slender, often long, and the body is thin with narrow shoulders and broad hips.

These are people who literally shine in the dark They can grasp ideas quickly, but they do not have the stamina to put these ideas across. This is part of their karma which has been brought over from past lives. They do not take care of their bodies and they eat little, thus making their bodies look fragile and delicate. The phosphorus people are the mind people, and they make good teachers, lecturers, and students of almost any subject their minds are put to. But they have the problem of a lack of balance of phosphorus. The body must have a normal intake of phosphorus to aid in calcium assimilation to maintain normal health.

The phosphorus people need a well-balanced diet, prescribed by someone who knows how to handle such problems. They also need a quiet atmosphere, recreation, and much sleep. They cannot take drugs and expect to keep in good health. Their greatest karma is the problem of thinking too much! They theorize, compare, imagine, analyze, speculate, and invent. This is good, but at the same time, it is not good when overdone, for it wears down the body's resistance to disease.

We are dealing in this chapter with astral circumstances and situations. These are the hidden factors of human existence, and they must become part of the knowledge of all who are interested in knowing about themselves and in gaining spiritually.

The karmic pattern of the individual is hardly anything more than astral and mental problems, especially the astral activities, the feeling and grasping areas within one's self. In the thousands of years man has been on this earth, he has hardly gone any further than the Astral Plane in his advancement.

The Astral is the plane of emotions. It is where the culture of the world exists, which includes the arts:

133

painting, music, writing, and sculpture. It is the plane of sentimental love, often mistaken for spiritual love. One has to take all of this into consideration when trying to work out some of his inner problems, especially when they are due to karmic patterns of past lives.

The *sulfur type* of person is handsome, with golden, reddish, or brown wavy hair. They have high foreheads and attractive smiles. Most of them are slender and talented in some artistic field, perhaps music, art, or writing. They are keenly interested in everything and very susceptible to luxuries, but their basic karma is an explosive temperament, and they expect all people to forgive them immediately. This sort of temper is also the cause of their skin troubles. A diet high in sulfur from raw foods would assist in their temperamental, sensitive problems; cooking foods changes the sulfur availability. They must also be careful of elimination conditions.

The *calcium-phosphorus* people are very delicate, refined, and extremely cultured. They have dark brown hair, slender necks, and somewhat poor vitality. Their heads are usually narrow and flat in the back, at the point where the spine joins the head.

The phosphorus in this type is generally burned up by great mental activity, making them nervous people. Without enough phosphorus for the rest of the body, the other minerals cannot be assimilated and used. Therefore, the calcium needed for the bones is not available. Lack of exercise in this type, because they like to read so much, keeps the oxygen supply low, so that the potassium which is present in the diet

134

cannot be used in the body. It is because of the potassium that iron becomes a part of the blood; without it the body becomes anemic, the person nervous and exhausted. This is part of the karma with this type of person.

Since the blood is not purified because of the low supply of oxygen, weak circulation and poor digestion result. If one gets enough exercise, this situation in his health condition can be remedied. The calcium-phosphorus type also has a great need for vitamins and requires more calcium foods with which to combat anemia. Also, nerve foods should be in the diet, such as raw eggs, coconut, and olives. This type of person should strike a balance between mental and physical exercise, get plenty of sunlight, and take deep breathing exercises and body massage.

This type should be careful not to deplete himself of what energies he already has. Being overactive can leave him depleted, and he should practice moderation in everything he does.

The last chemical category is called the *balanced type*. This is a combination of the calcium, carbon, and sulfur chemicals in the body. Calcium gives them strength of bones; carbon keeps the type congenial; and sulfur gives them a good appearance. The hair of this type is generally light brown or reddish, or they may be blonde with blue eyes.

One of the karmic patterns which they have is a weak digestion. They are thinkers who are active, as well as having good perception and insight into human nature. Reason, will, and logic all blend perfectly in this type. These are the ones who set their

135

goal for success and wealth in this material world and succeed.

If the sulfur aspect is greater than the others, that is, if it is out of balance, these individuals will have tempers which can explode without rhyme or reason. They can, also, even though balanced, outrun their natural energies and become depleted and have a poor oxygen intake because of a lack of exercise.

The balanced type must have a plain diet for his daily fare. He cannot eat desserts, rich pastries, or candies. If he begins to fall off this daily fare, then his health will start going down until he is unable to perform with efficiency.

One must begin to think about himself in terms of chemistry in his body according to minerals. We must remember that the mineral-rich person is a happy one and often very successful in his work. He radiates a personality so different and unusual that he is often admired instantly by those meeting him for the first time.

So many minerals of various types are needed by the body to provide health and the enjoyment of life, and they should never be overlooked. Those who understand these needs and how minerals influence the body are indeed blessed, because they can have longevity, work out many of their karmic problems, and have a wonderful spiritual unfoldment.

Since one's pattern of life can be judged from his birth into this world, at least some knowledge should be given so that each person can understand himself a little better.

What we are today is, of course, what our karma has made us; but on the other hand, there are so many factors in life and so many aspects to reincarnation and karma that it becomes nearly impossible to explain them to a lay reader. However, karma is a matter which can be cleared up in a relatively reasonable time, provided any individual wants to be rid of the heavier problems which confront him. Much of it can be done through the right approach to body health and in understanding the chemistry of the temple in which we each are enclosed in this world.

There will be arguments about this, and one of them is that if one has developed spiritually, none of these things are necessary. This is true, but how many spiritually developed people does one find in this world? How many come anywhere near the degree of perfection designated by the religionists and true spiritual giants? There are only a handful in comparison to the masses of people who have lived in the body since the beginning of time.

For example, supposedly there are ten billion people who have lived on earth since the time of Tiberius, the Roman emperor who reigned when Jesus lived and died. Of all these men and women who lived and died, nearly all have been forgotten. Only a few names remain on the pages of our history books. Of the names we know well, most are military conquerors; perhaps a handful are holy men, saviors, and mystics. Many of the latter lived only a short span of years. Some were murdered; others died in accidents. Still others lived a natural life span. In the case of Jesus, it was calculated assassination. Buddha died an accidental death, and Mohammed died of old age. But we find that only a few can be considered above the average man in spiritual development.

Few have ever caught the secret to good health, longevity, and spiritual perfection; since these three aspects of life are the result of an order and procedure of spiritual enlightenment that eventually yields God-Realization, it is not very likely that too many people are going to have them. But the fortunate ones do realize how they have been chosen to receive these gifts of God and are extremely thankful.

When we look at the lives of the ECK Masters, some of whom are beyond the age of normal man, it is daunting to try to understand the meaning of their long lives. These are Souls who have kept their original bodies on earth. The trio who are well known in Eckankar are Rebazar Tarzs, Fubbi Quantz, and Yaubl Sacabi. They have retained the original bodies which they took as Souls in this lifetime so very long ago.

Rebazar Tarzs, the youngest, is said to be some five hundred years old. This would mean that he came into this life during the fifteenth century and still occupies the same body today. The purpose of his keeping the physical body is that he was the Living ECK Master for quite some time before passing the Rod of ECK Power to another. He still retains his body although he lives practically in seclusion in a remote section of the Hindu Kush mountains. He was born in a western province of China, near Chamdo, on the border of Tibet.

Fubbi Quantz is the next oldest in the line of ECK Masters in the Ancient Order of Vairagi, which is the order of these particular Adepts. He is the head of the Katsupari Monastery in the Thanglha Mountains in northern Tibet where he has charge of a number of persons who are studying the works of ECK. He is also in charge of the first section of the Shariyat-Ki-Sugmad, the sacred scriptures of the ECK Masters.

Heading the order of the ancient ECK Masters is Yaubl Sacabi, who is the spiritual leader of the spiritual city of Agam Des, which is located among the remote crags of the Hindu Kush in the same area as Tirich Mir, one of the highest peaks in the world. It is located on the border between Afghanistan and Pakistan.

Few ever visit the spiritual city of Agam Des except by invitation. Its leader, Yaubl Sacabi, heads up the whole order of the ECK Masters on this planet, and his age is beyond human conception. He lives in the physical body much of the time, as do some of those who are citizens of this spiritual community. They use the famed drill of the *Eshwar Khanewale* (the God-eaters) to maintain their health and strength in the human body. They are able to consume the Cosmic Spirit for food, which preserves their bodies, enabling them to serve the inhabitants of the many planets in this universe. The second section of the Shariyat-Ki-Sugmad, located in the Temple of Golden Wisdom, is also under the guardianship of Yaubl Sacabi.

Anyone fortunate enough to learn rejuvenation methods, such as the *Ayur Vedha* system of renewing the body health, can look and feel thirty years younger. The *Kaya Kalp* treatment, which is a part of the Ayur Vedha method, is used mainly to bring back youth and health to anyone who is able to find it.

Before the Chinese invasion of Tibet, many of the Easterners who knew about the works of Eckankar, made pilgrimages to the Katsupari Monastery to undergo these youth and health treatments. Now the frontier has been blocked on the Tibetan border and few ever get across, unless they go the difficult way, risking life and limb, up through the mountain passes which have not yet been fully opened to traffic.

Among the things which are frowned upon by the ECK Masters is sweet chocolate. It is not recommended for the body health, especially in the form of candy. Yet today most of the candies and sweets, including desserts, are made from a chocolate base. It is found to be hard on the digestive system and should not be eaten.

The ECK Masters may eat a little solid food in public while in the presence of their followers — they might take bread, some meat, and tea. They will not try to act differently in order to arouse the curiosity of the people around them nor to attract attention. In fact, they will keep public attention away from themselves as much as possible. This is why they are often inaccessible and cannot be reached by the public.

People long for the ECK Master and will try to touch his hand, be near him, and gather to themselves anything possible from him. They will try to see him merely for *Darshan* (to receive a blessing by gazing upon his countenance). The ECK Master seldom gives thought to himself, his body, or to his needs here in the physical environment. Herbs, minerals, and plants are a natural part of the world which God has given man to keep his body healthy. The Living ECK Master will try in every way possible to attain and to increase his knowledge of all things, including health, nutrition, and foods for man in his journey to God.

7

The Sacred Herbs of the Ancient Mystics

More than a thousand years before the birth of Christ, a people known as the Shang, or Yin, lived along the Yellow River in north central China. Very little is known about their origin and history but their civilization was very old and very rich. They left abundant evidence of great technical skill in casting bronze, in shaping pottery, and in fashioning the written words which are the direct ancestors of the modern Chinese characters. From the inscriptions on bone and bronze, the names of some of their kings and the nature of their divination are known.

However, the greatest body of knowledge which these ancients left was their understanding of herbs. They spoke about ginger and other herbs, which are known today among the average Chinese, but their finest contribution was the ginseng plant. The ginseng grew wild in seclusion, hiding itself from man, seeking unfrequented deep, shady forests and hillsides for its growth.

The taste of *ginseng* is similar to that of licorice. The ancient Chinese developed it in accordance with their belief in its extraordinary virtue as an elixir of life. They used it as a remedy for many diseases, as well as for relief from the fatigue of the body and the mind. Today, the demand for the ginseng root in China is so great that large quantities are imported from other countries to keep up with the amount consumed by the Chinese people.

Ginseng is the common name for two species of the *Panax* herb, which comes from the *Araliaceae* family. The root of this herb provides the substance which is supposedly good for many ailments and for general health in China. The *Panax quinquefolius* is the American ginseng, which is a native plant of the cool woods of eastern North America, ranging southward to Florida, Alabama, Louisiana, and Arkansas. There is a vast amount of ginseng cultivated in America, most of which is carefully dried and exported to Hong Kong. From there it is distributed throughout Southeast Asia and China.

The Asiatic ginseng is native to Manchuria, Korea, and Japan. It is cultivated in large quantities there and sold throughout Asia, because it is often believed to be of a better quality than the American ginseng.

From time immemorial, the Chinese have believed that ginseng is a cure for all diseases and infirmities. The word *ginseng* is said to mean "the wonder of the world," while panax is from the Greek for "panacea." Because of its slow growth, it takes about five to seven years for the ginseng plant to mature from seed to the full plant, and the cultivation of ginseng as a plant is often confined to an acre for growing. Not too many people are interested in a harvest unless the crops are rotated so that there will be one each year.

This brings up an interesting point. According to history, which molds thoughts from generation to generation, the discovery of America benefited only Spain. This is not true, for it was the discovery of new plants, herbs, and other types of food products that revitalized Europe and the rest of the world.

The gold which poured out of the New World into the coffers of the Spanish kings was nothing in comparison to the nutritional wealth gained by the discovery of America. But at that time, few people, except for enterprising merchants, knew what was happening to their countries.

Christopher Columbus, who was a student of the ECK Master Fubbi Quantz, was encouraged to take his sea voyage to the West. Fubbi Quantz knew what was in store for the navigator, and he was very anxious for Columbus to make a sea journey in order to open up the new worlds beyond the Atlantic.

Fubbi Quantz was traveling through Europe at the time and was greatly impressed by the nutritional poverty of that continent's people. They were protein poor, and they needed a flood of the right products in order to overcome this condition. He knew that it took too long for ships to sail around the Cape of Good Hope to bring food to Europe.

Therefore, Fubbi Quantz saw no other solution than to open the doors of the Americas where the real gold of the Indies was the green products. From the new continent would come maize, the potato, the tomato, and legumes to ease the starvation diet of the European poor and to give them the protein needed for new energies. Man's life span in the fifteenth century was barely more than thirty-five years.

The new varieties of beans would ease the fasting of the clergy, for the kind of beans they had then were of the cattle-food type, the poorest protein type which could be found. Even the poor of India had food somewhat better than the European clergymen.

The American herbs and plants would go far toward helping to abolish poverty and to make the population more stable. They would provide the human energy for the changes of the industrial revolution and the new age of urbanization, and would enable the farmers and peasants — a small fraction of the population — to provide food for the rest of the European nations.

Fubbi Quantz, in the interest of humanity, laid out the plans for Columbus one evening in Genoa, in a vision similar to the one which George Washington had at Valley Forge during the winter of 1777. It was then that Columbus began to make known his plans for finding a new trade route to the East. He finally came to the court ruled by Ferdinand and Isabella, who were in need of something to bolster their economy. Although Ferdinand was reluctant, the Queen aided Columbus to outfit a fleet for his explorations. The discovery of the Western Hemisphere, with all its green gold, changed the face of the world, although none realized this at the time.

The Chinese claimed that their sick took ginseng to recover their health, while those in good health used it to make themselves resistant to disease. It is said that it is common for many Chinese women over seventy years of age, who are users of ginseng, to have children.

It is believed that the first knowledge of the medicinal herbs was written by a monk, Shun-Chung Tsang, in about the year 3100 B.C. Fragments of this manuscript have been found and recorded. Ginseng was regarded as the highest among the many herbs which were then in use and was used as a tonic to strengthen the body, prolong life, invigorate the mind, and for helping the romance of the heart.

Other references to ginseng have been noted here and there in the Chinese writings. Marco Polo found it in great use when he traveled through China during the year 1275. After a study of it, he did not believe that ginseng rated much interest, and he never had much to say other than noting that it was widely used among the Chinese for practically everything.

The reason wild ginseng sells for a much higher price than cultivated ginseng is that it is more potent and more difficult to secure. The belief that radioactive substances from the earth are more potent in ground where the ginseng grows wild also brings a better price for the wild plant. However, wild ginseng is more difficult to find, for it is believed that the ginseng plant is so sensitive that it will, at the slightest sound, fold its flowers and make itself look like other plants. Therefore, the ginseng hunter cannot readily detect it as he can other herbs and plants.

In Tibet, ginseng is found mostly in the northern areas where the natives gather the plants in the highlands. This is done during the early season of the year, right after the snow has left the ground and flowers and plants are springing up in profusion. The monks from the monasteries and the natives seek out the ginseng plant in the dark hollows of the hills where it hides itself from human eyes.

It is strange that ginseng is so highly regarded by the Oriental countries while at the same time it is almost entirely ignored by the West. Western health authorities have apparently not yet found any significant use for the ginseng plant. At the same time, the Russians have been doing an enormous amount of scientific research in learning about the herb.

During World War II, the Russian government had huge fields of ginseng growing in the wildest parts of the Sikhote-Alin Mountains. It was here that Russia placed several experimental stations and proved that the roots of the ginseng plant contained many radioactive properties. Now it is said that the Russians are still working with ginseng in south Siberia, where large plantations of ginseng have been planted, at a cost of millions of dollars to the government. So far, they have kept their findings secret and are not letting the rest of the world know why they are going into such tremendous research on the ginseng plant.

It is believed that the action of ginseng on the endocrine glands gives the body the power to make better use of vitamins and minerals, which helps to overcome nutritional deficiencies. The Greeks believed that ginseng had magical virtues. The Japanese think of it as a longevity herb, and the American Indians used it for stomach disorders.

Another herb plant which has collected mysteries and myths around itself is the *mandrake*. Its uses and

146

influence are given in most occult literature. It was one of the favorite plants of the magicians, for it is supposed to have powerful influences when used in magic spells and rituals.

The European mandrake is sometimes known as mandragora or Satan's apple. The mandrake belongs to the potato family. It is native to the temperate regions of the Mediterranean and the Himalayas. In ancient times the plant was dedicated to Circe, the enchantress, who was celebrated for her witchcraft. Ulysses, the wanderer, had an unpleasant encounter with mandrake during his voyage homeward following the Trojan wars.

Books by the score could be written about the lore of the mandrake plant. Mandrake was used by the ancient sorcerers for love philters, and it is mentioned in the Old Testament as an ingredient for love potions. In the Dark Ages, it is said that the roots of the mandrake were a part of the concoction put into the witch's cauldron. In the Middle Ages, a concoction of the mandrake was used as an opiate, as well as a love potion. It could have had the dual effect of putting one person to sleep, while stimulating another. It was common knowledge that during the Middle Ages the mandrake was supposed to grow under the gallows of hanged men. Pulled from the earth, the root gave out wild shrieks, and those who heard them were said to go insane.

The mandrake was said to be "the dragon which resembles man," and there is supposedly a female and male form, each looking so much like the two sexes of man that it is amazing. The way the roots sometimes wrapped around one another, it appears as if one plant were symbolic of a woman, and another, a man. The ancient magicians and priests believed that it was the root of creation. It was thought that the ancient Japanese sorcerers actually created life by manipulating the mandrake roots, then breathing life into them.

It is claimed by the old magicians that if anyone would pull up the mandrake root at midnight, in the light of the full moon, then clean it and write the name of his beloved upon it, she would never leave him for another. Or if he would write whatever was his greatest desire in life, it would come true.

Of course, there were many other types of spells which the magicians used—for example, those that would bring money, improved health, mental stimulation, and fruitful crops. There are supposed to be no less than twenty-five different types of mandrake-based spells that the magician may utilize for his clientele.

I seriously warn against anyone swallowing mandrake because of its poisonous properties. Alone or when mixed with other ingredients, the mandrake can be highly dangerous to the human body. Mandrake has been banned by the U.S. government and cannot legally be sold in the United States.

Carob, or St. John's bread, is the fruit of the carob tree. Finely ground, it takes the place of cocoa, chocolate, and to some extent, sugar. It contains a sufficient amount of vitamins and minerals to qualify as one of the worthwhile plants which can be considered here. It is actually an evergreen tree of the pea family, *Leguminosae.*

148

It is a native of the eastern Mediterranean area. It grows to about thirty feet in height and has numerous branches, forming a rounded head with shining dark leaves, which have two or three pairs of leaflets. Its flowers are in small red clusters with numerous brown, hornlike, flat pods, which are from six to twelve inches long, one to one and one-half inches broad, and a quarter of an inch thick. The pods contain many hard, small, dark brown seeds, which are imbedded in a sweet, mealy, edible pulp. These pods are dark brown in color, rich in natural sugar, protein, and B vitamins.

The hard seeds are removed from the pod, and the pod is toasted to increase the flavor. Then it is ground into a fine powder which is used as a substitute for chocolate or cocoa in beverages, candies, cookies, and as a general flavoring. Carob does not contain any of the stimulants or harmful factors that chocolate contains. Many who are allergic to chocolate, cocoa, and milk, use carob instead.

The carob pods are important for food and forage. Mohammed's armies on the march sometimes lived on kharub, or what we know as carob. The ancient Romans, Spaniards, and British all knew the carob tree and lived on its pods when other food was scarce. John the Baptist ate the carob pod in the wilderness, so it is said, giving it the appellation, St. John's Bread.

Carob is used for animal feed. The wood is used for staining, and the roots contain medicinal properties. The grown tree can yield up to one thousand pounds of pods in a season. It is exceedingly productive, and there are orchards of carob trees in the warm climate states of America such as California, Florida, and Texas.

Medicinally, carob is a mild laxative and demulcent. Some singers use the carob pod husks in the belief that it clears their voice and helps their throat. Gum is extracted from the seeds and used in various industries such as textile, pharmaceutical, food, leather, rubber, and cosmetics. Carob gum is imported from several European countries.

Carob may replace the starchy sweets that we have learned to crave in this civilization. The refined sugar, which goes into so many of the sweets in our national food diet, is not at all good for body health, while carob contains many vitamins and minerals. The body must take its good health out of everything which is given it. Unless every bite contains vitamins and minerals, it is harmful to burden the body with it. Carob contains thiamine (B_1), that important B vitamin so necessary for the proper digestion of carbohydrates. Thiamine is also essential for the good health of the nerves which, of course, makes for good morale. Carob also contains a good amount of niacin, another B vitamin which is responsible for the health of the digestive tract. Another B vitamin in carob is riboflavin (B_2), which is needed for the health of the skin and eyes.

Carob contains carotene which the body uses to produce vitamin A, the fat soluble vitamin which protects the eyes from night blindness and infections. It also contains calcium, phosphorus, iron, and magnesium. It is not necessary that carob be in the daily diet, but it can be a staple and should be used in place of candy, if needed to satisfy a child's desire for sweets.

150

Of course, carob is not the full answer to the needs of the bodily intake of the B vitamins. We get more of this vitamin in meat, fish, and poultry, according to most authorities. Animal protein is a complete protein, which contains more essential amino acids than vegetable protein.

Meat is a high quality protein, rich in iron and the B vitamins, especially riboflavin and niacin. In the milling of grains, many of the B vitamins are lost. The use of meats in the diet provides these essential vitamins that are nonexistent in the devitalized processed food so prevalent today.

Americans are a meat-eating people. In fact, most of the Occidentals are, and if they were not, they would be in bad health because of the excessive use of processed starches and sugars in the national diets.

Goldenseal is one of the old herbs used by the natives and ancients in many countries throughout the world. However, we mainly find it among the Indian tribes of North America, who once relied on it almost entirely for many of their medical needs. Not having the science of medicine as we do today, the North American primitives had to depend wholly upon the plant and herb kingdom for their medicinal needs. This was natural, and it has brought much of their findings into our research laboratories today so that we might understand just what the Indians had that helped them to keep their health under such primitive conditions. Goldenseal was one of their favorite herbs. The natives of early New England settlements soon learned to use goldenseal for medicinal purposes. The name goldenseal was given to this plant

151

because of the seal-like scars on the golden yellow roots.

In the southeastern United States, the Cherokee tribe made great use of this marvelous little herb. The people used it as a remedy for sore mouths, inflamed eyes, and as a bitter tonic in stomach and liver disorders. They also employed it externally for diseases of the skin, and it became very popular among the early settlers. The fresh root is quite juicy, and it was used by the Indians as a dye for their garments and as a stain for faces during rituals and ceremonies.

Sometimes the goldenseal is called yellow root, tumeric root, or Indian paint. It is native to Canada and the eastern United States. It belongs to the buttercup family. The Indians of North America used the plant originally as a dye and a sort of cosmetic. The tea brewed from the roots of the plant contains several valuable alkaloids of which hydrastis is the most important. Hydrastis is a bitter crystalline, nonpoisonous alkaloid found in the rootstock of the goldenseal and used as a tonic. Its action is tonic, laxative, and alterative. It is a valuable remedy in digestive conditions, and it has a local, corrective effect on the mucous membranes, especially in the inflammation of the colon and rectum.

The root of the goldenseal, known scientifically as *Hydrastis canadensis,* is a bright yellow color and is crooked and wrinkled. In the center of two rough leaves appears the flower, which is displaced by the large-seeded berry. The root is used in the treatment of leucorrhea, inflammation of the bladder, and as a tonic to refresh and invigorate the muscular system of the body.

During the early part of the nineteenth century, medical authorities began to experiment with the goldenseal root because of historical reports of its usefulness. Accounts of the benefits of goldenseal had been handed down from generation to generation, mostly by word of mouth about the Indian remedies. The Indians used it as strong tea for indigestion, low fevers, and for cases of general weakness. It was also used as a wash for inflammation of the eyes. Hydrastis, the product of the goldenseal root, was given a careful review of its properties, uses, and preparations by the medical laboratories. As a result, it was declared an official drug in the pharmacopoeia of this country in 1860, and a great demand was created through its new uses.

In these modern times, goldenseal has become quite useful to the botanic industry in modern preparations. It is used in preparations for the eyes, such as eye drops and eye washes, as hydrastis is one of the chief ingredients in such medicines. It is also used in morning sickness, sore mouth and eyes, eczema, indigestion, and catarrh. Some medical authorities use it in their practices, so it is said, as a stimulating tonic in cases of indigestion and gastric debility, and for the nervous system. (For more on goldenseal, see chapter 4.)

Goldenrod, like goldenseal, contains a bright yellow dye, but there is no other connection between the two plants. Goldenseal is a little plant growing near the ground while goldenrod is often three feet tall with a tuft of small golden blossoms on the top like a thousand little tassels. It blooms in late summer and can be very impressive. It is a plant which lends its

153

color to the beauty of the countryside in the autumn of the year. Late in the year when the blooms have gone to seed, it can be dipped in old oil and burned like a torch.

The flowers and tops of the goldenrod are used to make a valuable kidney and bladder remedy. Goldenrod is also used as an antiseptic.

This plant is often called Aaron's rod, woundwort, and goldruth, to name a few. It has long been famous for healing wounds when used externally and as an infusion when taken internally. It has diuretic properties, and it has an excellent and time-honored reputation for dissolving kidney stones and for ulcer pains. Goldenrod leaves make a rather pleasant, aromatic tea.

The ancients used it for many of the above purposes, while in the modern age it has been used as an astringent.

The goldenrod belongs to the *Compositae* family, the largest of all plant families. It grows in a great variety of places like woods, meadows, hills, and rocky ground. Goldenrod was for a long time believed to be a cause of hayfever but experiments have proven that ragweed is the major culprit.

Goldenrod is a perennial herb with several species, many of them native to North America, but it originally was discovered in the ancient days in the Middle East. Traditionally it sprouted from Aaron's rod when he threw his staff upon the ground before the Pharaoh to demonstrate his magic.

All these herbs seem to have played a definite part in the lives of the ancient mystics. Furthermore, they have had something to do with the evolution of man

154

in the course of history. Every plant and herb which has added some assistance to man's health problems by curing him of some ailment, disease, or sickness, is considered a part of the growth of the human race.

There are indications that diagnosis by computer and electronic apparatus today may not get to the real source of trouble in the human body and mind. Psychosomatic problems, which include depression, irritability, anxiety, fears, difficulties in concentration, short memory span, uncontrollable weeping, insomnia, fatigue, inability to make decisions, sensitivity to slight noises, and ferocious temper tantrums complicated by nightmares, shortness of breath, dizziness, blurred vision, and thoughts of suicide, can be due to a lack of a proper diet.

There is always a reason for what is happening to the body, and no one should expect a cure, healing, or a miracle to take place in his health after twenty-five years of bad nutrition. He created his own problem, and he must bear the responsibility for it.

I will go back again to the problem of fasting, which many of those who are of a religious mind do not fully understand. Those who undertake a prolonged fast may lose a few teeth, peace of mind, and the ability to resist infection. These conditions are created when, and if, the individual who is going on such a fast has not prepared himself with plenty of vitamin B_6.

Those who fast may find themselves unable to enjoy their new portion of religious visions and the broadening of their outlook on life, because they have become too tense, irritable, and unable to sleep. They could also find themselves suffering oily skin, dandruff, and acne. These are the manifestations of a deficiency of vitamin B_6. This particular vitamin is necessary to the health of the skin and gums, the utilization of fats, the building of the blood, and the action of the muscles.

These are common symptoms found in studying the records of those religious figures who did so much fasting in order to gain some experiences of God. It has also been demonstrated by health authorities that a deficiency of vitamin B_6 does develop during prolonged fasts and that specific manifestations may result.

It is not exactly that fasting alone will cause a deficiency of vitamin B_6, for even a poor diet can bring about nervousness, insomnia, general weakness, and sometimes difficulty in walking. Even in the midst of plenty, where poor nutrition is not necessary, the same tendencies in the human mind and body are found. As much as eighty percent of the essential amino acid tryptophan is destroyed when vitamin B_6 is not properly supplied.

The individual should be certain about his health before attempting a prolonged period of fasting. Only if one is in fairly good health can he have the necessary religious experiences. One should balance his nutritional life with other aspects of daily living.

The old religionists who were able to fast knew quite a bit about their personal intake of food and what gave them particular problems and what did not. They could sometimes go without food for days.

Today, although food is bountiful and there are relatively few people starving in the Western world, people may not be as aware of their nutritional problems and therefore have more difficulty in emulating the ancient religionists.

The mystics have played their part on the stage of mankind by their acute knowledge of plants and herbs, which not only helped with the nutritional value of diets for man, but also has assisted in his general health, keeping him well and fit to make his cities and country a better place to live.

8

The Strange and Curious Herbs
That Bring Health

Some readers may have wondered what the philosophy and doctrine of Eckankar, the Ancient Science of Soul Travel, has to do with herbs, plants, and general health-giving foods.

The spiritual philosophy of Eckankar contends that the body should have good health in order to have a better life while here on earth. Pain is never pleasant, regardless of what age one is or under what circumstances he may suffer. Should a person be willing to suffer pain for the sake of his religious doctrine, well and good, but few can live in this world and still strive for spiritual understanding in ill health.

This book does not propose to replace the services of anyone's family physician. One should always consult him for any condition which requires his services. But the individual should take the responsibility for trying to keep himself in good health. He must learn something about nutrition and what his body chemistry can handle in the way of foods, herbs, and fruits.

The health and life-giving herbs, plants, flowers, and fruits have something to do with one aspect of ECK, and that is in the general area of health and healing.

Eckankar has thirty-two facets, among which two are of interest here. First, is the eighteenth facet, known as the banishing of pain and pleasure. This is part of the health and healing program which is under discussion in this book. Second, is spiritual healing, which is the twenty-seventh facet. I will touch upon spiritual healing here and there throughout the rest of the book.

We find that this ECK herb book is only one in the whole line of the spiritual works of Eckankar. Each of the thirty-two facets, discussed somewhat in *The ECK Satsang Discourses,* First Series, will be covered sooner or later in the books which will be published on the overall subject of Eckankar.

In taking up the study of those strange and curious plants and herbs which give health to the mind and body of the individual, we are struck by the fact that so many of them seem to have been neglected by modern research, yet the generations of the past appear to have benefited from their use of them for general health.

The first we shall consider is the *Eglantine,* commonly known as sweetbriar. It is a part of the rose family known to science as *Rosa rubiginosa.* It is a dense shrub often six feet tall and its stem bears hooked thorns. The top side of the leaf is dark green;

the underside is much lighter in color and has a pleasant aromatic coating. The flowers are bright pink and sweet scented. The fruit is orange-red or scarlet.

The eglantine is native to Europe, especially the central European countries. It has been widely used in gardens because of its pleasant scent.

The rosebuds ripen into a fruit called hips, which are dried, and a tea is made from them. The hip tea is good for purifying the kidneys and bladder. Those who have kidney stones can take a cup of this tea each day to help resolve the irritants in the kidneys and bladder.

Cloves are the dried flower buds of the clove tree. Sometimes called spice clove, it is a part of the family of myrtles. The clove tree grows from fifteen to thirty feet high. It is an evergreen with a trunk measuring four to six feet which soon divides into large branches rising to form a pyramid. The wood is hard and tough so that quite small branches will bear the weight of a man. The bark is somewhat smooth and bare. The leaves are lanceolate, narrow and pointed. They are smooth and glossy green on top and velvety, light greenish-brown on the bottom. The flowers are very small in large clusters and have an exotic fragrance. The tree is beautiful in every respect and is pleasant to sit under anytime of the year because of its delicate perfume.

The flowers are small, but bloom in great profusion in cymes. The leaves, flowers, and bark have an aromatic odor. The ripe fruit resembles an olive in shape, but is smaller in size. When allowed to mature most of its pungency is lost.

The flower buds are the principal products of the tree. They are gathered and are dried by exposure to the smoke of wood fires or to the sun's rays. When first gathered, they are reddish, but they change to a deeper brown color. Clove is a native of the Spice Islands, but is now cultivated in Sumatra, the East and West Indies, Brazil, and Guinea.

The properties of cloves depend chiefly on an essential oil known as oil of cloves, which forms one-fifth of the total weight. The oil obtained from the clove is sold by pharmacies; it is also used as the base of many different patent medicines. From four to six drops of oil of cloves on a piece of sugar taken once or twice a day is a good remedy for stomach gases. Clove oil is also used for toothache, and, because of its antiseptic properties and pleasant taste, to flavor dentifrices. Being one of the least expensive essential oils, clove is also used in industrial perfumery; for example, in the scenting of soaps. The herb, of course, is used for cooking and seasoning.

The *elder,* or the black elder or common elder, as it is sometimes called, is a shrub or tree which grows from ten to thirty feet high.

It is an herb that is used quite commonly by many who are living in the less civilized areas of the central European countries. The farm people and many who live in the country have used it for generations.

The bark of the trunk is light brown or gray, and rough. The branches are smooth with distinct wart-like bumps. The white, hard wood has a whitish pith at the center. The leaves consist of two and three pairs of leaflets, long and tapering at the base, long-

162

pointed at the extremity, serrated, dark green, and hairless. The flowers are white or pale yellow and wheel-shaped. The berries grow to the size of peas, or smaller, and are dark violet or reddish and juicy.

The elder is a good spring tonic, according to an old German herbal formula which calls for the fine cutting of six to eight leaves to be simmered for ten minutes in a cup of water. A cup of this herbal water should be drunk before and after breakfast. It can be used at any time of the year and prepared from dried leaves if necessary.

The same German source says that a tea can be made from the flowers of the elder shrub which will produce a good remedy for dropsy.

A tablespoon of the elder berries boiled in sugar or honey and stirred into a glass of water will make a refreshing drink, clearing the stomach of gases and undigested foods, acting as a stimulant to the kidneys for diuretic purposes.

Another old German herbal formula calls for boiling the dried berries to a pulp, simmering them into a tea, or eating them dry for a beneficial effect in case of severe diarrhea. One should remember that these are old German formulas for health, and he should obtain the advice of someone who knows the benefits of a treatment, instead of depending upon remedies handed down through generations.

The elder is a mild herb that can be used freely with little danger. It is used with mint to break up congestion from colds and flu. Taken warm after a long hot bath, it is said to stop or shorten a cold. Used with peach bark it is a good diuretic and will help remove excess water.

Elder berries grow in great clusters, and they are probably the easiest of all fruit to pick. The Indians would pick the dried fruit of the elder, pound the dried berries with dried meat and animal fat, and wrap the mixture in yellow dock leaves.

The *butterbur* is an herb which is a native of Europe. The flower stalk is about six to eighteen inches in height and as thick as a man's finger. It is covered with gray hair and has a large triangular leaf that is pear-shaped at the base, smooth on the upper surface, and woolly gray beneath.

The flower is closely packed and oval. Its color is a purplish gray, and it is tubular in nature. A tea made from the root is used in clearing the chest and lungs of phlegm. It is also used for treating coughs and tightness of the throat and chest. Putting wet leaves on the chest is supposed to help reduce fever in consumption.

Saint-John's-wort is a plant which belongs to the Saint-John's-wort family called *Hypericaceae*. It is a native of the subtropical and temperate regions throughout the world, including Europe and the United States. Some species are widely cultivated in gardens, and St.-John's-wort also grows wild on dry heaths, plains, roadsides, ridges, and in forest clearings. There are over 300 species of St.-John's-wort, but we will mainly be dealing with St.-John's-wort (*Hypericum perforatum*).

It was named after John the Baptist during the Middle Ages by monks who developed gardens and were skilled in the medicinal use of herbs. The wort is said to blossom on St. John's eve and was believed to pos-

164

sess magical properties, such as protecting one against thunder and evil spirits. Various healing properties have been attributed to the different species of the plant, generally as an astringent, nervine, and expectorant.

The flowers are infused in olive oil and applied to wounds and bruises. Both the flowers and leaves are used for a tea to help liver complaints. In one old herbal remedy, it is said that the older generations used it for pains in the head arising from congestion or catarrh.

It is a perennial which grows about two feet high; the stems spring from one root with auxiliary branches. Saint-John's-wort bears an attractive yellow flower cluster. It is a popular garden flower used mainly for ornamental purposes.

The common Saint-John's-wort is the most abundant of the wild species and is known as a weed throughout the United States, as well as the rest of the world. The petals of its flowers are twice as long as the sepals and are golden yellow, dotted with black along the edges.

Shepherd's purse is a small shrub which was used as a medical remedy in Europe in earlier generations, and is still in use today among many who live in the rural areas.

It is a plant which grows about two feet high. The stem is straight, and its rosette of basal leaves are partly oblong and roughly serrated. The upper leaves are arrow-shaped and half embrace the stem with toothed margins. Its flowers are short, white, four-petaled, and small. The plant is long-stalked and the seed pods are triangular. It is easily recognized.

It is found throughout the world in fields, gardens, near homes, and on roadsides. It is especially abundant in the European countries where it originated.

Shepherd's purse flowers throughout most of the year, especially in countries where the winters are mild. Its leaves, flowers, and husks are all used in herbal remedies. By simmering the leaves in wine or by reducing them to a powder and mixing them with wine, the herb may be drunk whenever needed.

Shepherd's purse is also a powerful diuretic and was used as a remedy for intermittent fever with enlargement of the spleen or liver, and for complaints of the stomach. This remedy was made up of a half handful of flowers and seed pods boiled in three cups of water. A cupful of this was drunk when needed. The powder was also used for fresh wounds. It was supposed to have a powerful healing effect and stopped bleeding.

The *valerian* root is the proper herb to soothe and quiet the nerves when the nervous system is in a highly irritated condition.

The valerian is known by several other names— great wild valerian, German valerian, all-heal, amantilla, setwall, and English valerian. It is a native of Europe and northern Asia. It is found in woodlands, river banks, hedges, mostly in damp spots, but occasionally in dry spots and barren slopes. It flowers from June through September, depending mainly upon the climate where it grows. Usually, it flowers best in July in the northern Asiatic countries and earlier in European climates.

The valerian is noted for its roots, which give the herbal qualities for remedies. This root consists of numerous pointed, brown, closely-packed rootlets, white in the interior, with a peculiar, fetid odor. The stem grows about three feet high, upright, round, and is hollow with leaves in pairs. The leaves are pointed, narrow, and toothed. The flowers form a cyme and the fruit buds are adnate. The flowers are white and tubular with five blunt parts. The flowers are cut off as buds in order to encourage the root to grow.

The root alone is used and is generally dug in the fall, after the plant has finished its growth. The root is cut and dried, then stored or made into powder. It must be kept in an airtight container. It is useful in all sorts of nervous complaints, whether they consist of cramps, pains, headaches, or stomach gases.

Its medicinal action and uses are anodyne, nervine, and antispasmodic. It may be used in all cases of nervous debility, so the herbal authorities state. It is also used in irritation of the nerves and in hysterical afflictions. It allays pain and promotes sleep. It is said to be a strong nervine without any narcotic effects, and valerian is used in various herbal, nervine, and antispasmodic compounds. It is said to be useful in epilepsy and convulsions. The valerian root is supposed to influence the circulation, slowing the heartbeat, increasing its strength. One caution: Excessive or extended use may produce headaches and symptoms of poisoning.

The *Oregon grape* is an herb which is common to the western coast of the United States and the Rocky Mountains. Its common names are mountain grape, holly-leaved barberry, California barberry, and mahonia. It is one of the best among the herbs for purifying the blood, as a tonic for the digestive system, and as a stimulant for the liver.

The Oregon grape is an evergreen shrub which grows to a height of approximately three to ten feet. It bears small yellow flowers with spiny, glossy, dark green leaves. Its flowers have six sepals, six petals, six stamens, and a solitary pistil. The fruit is an attractive, bluish-black berry. The plant is the state flower of Oregon, and it is cultivated as a hedge shrub in the United States.

The part used is the root. It is boiled in distilled water and taken orally for weak digestion, jaundice, blood impurities, and as a general tonic for the whole body system. It is said that the herbal remedy made from the root will restore health and increase strength and vitality to many who are suffering from a sluggish liver, weak stomach, indigestion, and sallow skin.

The *buckthorns* are shrubs found in the temperate and tropical regions of Europe, Asia, Africa, and the Americas. There are several different kinds of buckthorn, and several different herbal remedies are prepared from either the berries or bark. The name, buckthorn, comes from the spines on the ends of the branches of some species. The leaves are bright green and oval; the flowers are small, axillary, white, yellowish, or green, and clustered. These plants are sometimes cultivated in shrub borders.

Cascara sagrada, the California buckthorn, of the Pacific Coast of the United States is a tree fifteen to twenty feet high, the bark of which yields cascara sagrada, a laxative. The American Indian used this herb. It was called chittam bark. They would harvest it and store it in a leather sack high in the tepee for at least two years. This storage causes the herb to be much gentler in its laxative action.

The common buckthorn, a shrub native to England, has been naturalized in the United States and has round, blue-black berries about the size of a pea. From these berries a strong cathartic is made. A yellow dye is prepared from the bark.

The alder buckthorn is a shrub, sometimes called the black dogwood, frangula bark, and black alder dogwood. The alder buckthorn is a native of Europe and northern Asia. The medicinal action is purgative. It should be used with caution, never during pregnancy. Aging the bark for a year or more or heating to 212 degrees will gentle the action of the herb. It is used more now in veterinary practice.

Alder buckthorn was used as a tonic to cleanse the blood and stimulate the stomach and bowels. Other uses come from the berries, which were boiled in syrup and administered in small doses to serve as a strong purgative, according to an old mid-European herbal formula. Otherwise, buckthorn was given with honey to modify its taste, if so prescribed by a recognized herbal authority or the family physician.

The *passion flower* is a native of the West Indies and the southern part of the United States. It is what we call a mystical flower because it is traditionally associated with the crucifixion.

When the Spanish first found this flower growing wild in America, the priests called it the flower of passion, because its corona represented to them the crown of thorns they associated with the crucifixion.

169

Shortly after they came into this country, the Spanish sent the species back to Rome where it was cultivated and introduced into other countries.

It is a climber and is regarded as one of the most lovely plants used for covering trellises and arbors. There are several species, some of which produce fruits that can be eaten for food or made into juices in their native climes. As a climber, it often reaches the top of the highest trees where it is sustained by tendrils, producing an abundance of beautiful white and purple flowers.

The passion flower has small seeds and digitate leaves. Its medical ingredient was used in ancient herbal remedies as a sedative, antispasmodic, and nervine. It is still used in various parts of the world today for these particular elements in herbal remedies. It also is considered a reliable remedy in treating nervous disorders, insomnia, and hysteria. Some say that the herb is particularly effective in alleviating cases of occupational strain and severe mental stress, anxiety, and pressures of modern living.

In the United States, many of the sleeping pills and nerve sedatives sold in drug stores without a prescription contain the passion flower as one of their main ingredients. It is best to use professionally prepared formulas.

Shave grass is a plant whose natural habitat is North America, Eurasia, and Australia. It is found in fields and pastures and is common throughout the country, growing in all sorts of soil.

It has several different names — shave grass, horsetail grass, pewterwort, Dutch rushes, paddock pipes, and bottle brush. Only the herbaceous part of the herb, the green, barren shoots and the tails are used for any remedies.

It is a plant which grows about one to two feet in height; its branches are wiry and stiff, numerous and easy to pick off. These branches resemble the stiff hair of a horse's tail. There are several different species, but the quality of the branches is the same. Although some branches are arched and droopy, others are stiff and spreading, somewhat bent. Shave grass grows in segments one to four inches long which are easily separated. Children will pull them apart, bite off the large end, smash the small end with their teeth, and make a whistle out of it.

The medicinal action and uses are diuretic and astringent; it has been used to treat dropsy and kidney afflictions. A dram of the dried, powdered herb, taken three or four times a day, has also proved to be effective in halting the spitting of blood, so say certain herbalists. Shave grass is said to be one of the best herbs for the treatment of cystic ulcerations and ulcers of the urinary passages and hemorrhages.

Shave grass is also good as an emmenagogue. The plant will stop bleeding and assist in healing. It is sometimes used to reduce the swelling of eyelids and parts of the face. It is a very good source of silicon for a beautiful complexion. It is said to be used by the natives in the rural areas of the countries where it grows as a remedy for nosebleed.

The tea made from the herb is said to clear the stomach of gases and to help in the digestion of food. In the Middle Ages, it was used to heal wounds from battle action.

171

Balm is a common name for a fragrant, perennial herb in the mint family. It is native to Europe and grows wild on wooded mountains and in hedges and vineyards. It also has long been cultivated in gardens.

The plant grows from one to three feet in height. It is bushy and erect, with branches starting at the base. The leaves are grass green, rather heart-shaped, and the flowers, which blossom from July through September, are a light greenish white in color. Balm has a pleasant lemon-like scent.

The stems and leaves are still used occasionally in medicine as a gentle stimulant and tonic, and were once in great demand. The taste is somewhat astringent and the odor slightly aromatic.

The leaves are collected before the time of flowering, dried in the air, and are generally used in the form of tea, about one ounce to a half pint of water. The tea is drunk for body pains which arise from disturbances of the nervous system and for hysteria. Balm tea is also used for stomach cramps, digestive disturbances, and colic.

Balm was called melissa among the ancient Arabs and was cultivated in gardens and hedges. The physicians often recommended it for affections of the heart; in other words, it was a love potion. Paracelsus, the famous herbal physician of the Middle Ages, claimed the drinking of balm tea would bring about the complete rejuvenation of whoever used it. Because of this claim, balm was often steeped in wine and used as an ingredient in love potions and brews.

Balm is among many herbs which seem to have

been a part of the mythology of man. Curious legends have sprung up around balm.

Balm of Gilead is mentioned in the Bible a number of times. This balm comes from a small tree native to Arabia, the balsam of Gilead. A resin substance is taken from the trees and sold exclusively in Arabia and Asiatic countries today.

The *orange* is another product to be taken up here as a use for herbal and health remedies. Of course, it is a fruit and considered so, but the orange may be used in several different ways as a source of vitamin products, as in the vitamins A, B, and C and as a botanical for body health.

The orange is also called forbidden fruit and golden apple. There were certain writers of the ancient period of history who flatly stated that the orange was really the mythical golden apple of Hesperides. Greek mythology is filled with stories about these golden apples. It is said that Zeus gave Hera an orange when they married, and as a result, its blossoms have become a bridal flower in many countries, including the United States.

However, it is now being proven that the orange, as well as other citrus fruits, are important factors in the well-balanced diet. The orange possesses many valuable health and medicinal properties. The peeling of the orange was used during the twelfth century as a tonic by the Chinese. A fermentation of its flowers was a remedy for the heart, and the juice mixed with water was remedial for certain fevers.

The orange is a native of South China and Indochina. We find that the ancient Chinese writings refer to oranges as early as 2200 B.C. Columbus carried orange seeds for planting in the New World. Early in the sixteenth century, orange plantings were made in Mexico and Central America. Oranges were planted in Florida in 1565, and in Southern California in 1769.

Lemons, too, are considered very important in the all-around diet of man. The lemon has a somewhat broader use than the orange in the medicinal field. It is a native of the tropical regions of India and Burma, where it has grown wild since prehistoric times. It spread from Persia to Egypt and Palestine about the year 1000, and it finally was introduced into Spain by the Arabs in the twelfth century. Columbus brought the seeds to the West Indies from the Canary Islands in 1493, on his second trip to the New World. Since then it has spread to almost every tropical country in the world.

Lemons have been used in a variety of ailments, such as sore throat, colds, rheumatism, headaches, heartburn, upset stomach, hiccoughs, chapped lips, chilblains, and insect bites. The lemon was once used as a supplement to the diet of seafaring crews to ward off scurvy. At the present time, most of its medicinal use is for its vitamin C and bioflavonoids.

Other citrus fruits used for the health of the body are the grapefruit, lime, tangerine, and the pitanga, or Surinam cherry, of Brazil. The latter is a good source of calcium, phosphorus, and iron. Brazil has several other health fruits which are the pinguin, grumichama, jagua, and pitomba. All have good vitamin C content as well as iron, riboflavin, calcium, and enzymes that are useful to the body. They also have many other commercial uses.

Citrus fruits are high in calcium, high in sugar, and the acids are weak and easily broken down. So they act in the body as alkalizers rather than acidifiers. If the body chemistry is already alkaline (70 percent of the people have a tendency to be alkaline), citrus fruits should be used sparingly, as this can further upset the acid-alkaline balance. If alkalosis is a problem, use vinegar (apple cider vinegar) one to seven tablespoons per day in water and avoid citrus fruits. On the other hand, if you have a tendency toward acidosis, then citrus fruits could be very helpful in balancing this condition. Here we are referring to the pH of the urine. This is easily tested with pH tape available at a drug store. Your pH should be near six. If it is low as five then acidosis may be a problem. Seven and above indicates alkalosis.

Vervain, a member of the verbena family, is a plant which is native to Europe and Asia and naturalized across North America. It is found along roadsides and in dry grassy fields. Other names for it are enchanter's herb, holy herb, simpler's joy, and Juno's tears.

It has been, since the beginning of time, a symbol of enchantment. It is said that the ancient magicians and priests used this mystic herb in their divinations. Vervain was dedicated to Venus, the Goddess of Love, in practically every ritual. Even today it is still regarded as a plant which possesses power as a love philter.

It was a custom in the early days to steep the whole plant in water, which was then used for cleaning the house in order to keep away evil spirits. Another

175

belief was that by wearing a few leaves on the person, the vervain might protect one from harm.

Vervain is an herb common in most countries with temperate climates. It is not only a nervine, but also a tonic, antispasmodic, astringent, diaphoretic, and a diuretic. It will also correct, so it is stated, shortness of breath, wheezing, and circulatory weakness. Vervain is said to aid convalescence following illness and to give help to liver and spleen ailments.

One widely used herb is *boneset*. Its natural habitat is North America, growing in damp, swampy places, meadows, and on banks of small streams. It has long been recognized as a tea with a somewhat bitter flavor. Boneset was used by the settlers who, in the early days of this country, had to live in adverse conditions in log cabins with earthen floors, where it was cold, damp, and miserable. They used boneset tea as a nightcap to warm themselves, as well as a stimulant for their nerves.

The parts used in boneset are the dried leaves and the flowering tops. Boneset has several common names, such as thoroughwort, teasel, agueweed, feverwort, Indian sage, and sweating plant. It is versatile and used almost daily in herb remedies for a varied number of ailments. It is not only one of nature's greatest remedies for colds and fevers, but it is also known as a good tonic and antispasmodic.

The American Indians used it mainly to break the influenza fever, for boneset is said to take away both the ache and fever. Its therapeutic properties include, besides those named above, it being used as a diaphoretic, emetic, and aperient.

The *common sage,* sometimes called the sage of virtue and garden sage, is a small scrubby plant with branching stems, which often grow to the height of twelve to twenty-four inches. The stems bear numerous leaves and are four-sided. The entire plant is covered with a very short, gray down. The leaves are oblong, much wrinkled on the surface, deeply wrinkled on the underside, with a mid-rib and arch-shaped veins. The flowers are in numerous whorls on long spikes which terminate the branches. Sage flower is of a velvet blue color, a half-inch long.

The sage is found in wild, rocky, barren places in the southern Alps, in the Austrian Littoral, in the Canton Ticino (a part of southern Switzerland), and in Illyria. It grows wild in Germany, especially in the chalk districts where the plant has long been grown for domestic purposes.

Sage is cultivated in gardens all over the world. Its time for flowering is June and July. The leaves are usually gathered before the plant blooms, then dried and powdered. The flower is useless for any medicinal purposes, according to the European herbalists. Sage is used for bathing and dressing of long-standing open sores, and when it is used as a tea, will remove any discharge from the gums and throat. If the tea is mixed with wine and water, it purifies the liver and kidneys. Powdered sage sprinkled on food produces the same effect.

The ancients used it for seasoning food, which we follow today in herb cooking. It is an astringent, stimulant, and expectorant. It is recommended for liver complaints. A mixture of honey and sage was a remedy used for consumption in the old days. Sage is recommended by herbalists for rheumatism. Laced with lemon and honey and boiled in water, sage is said to have the power to ward off colds. It is easily grown in a garden from seed or transplanted roots. It is a perennial herb.

Fenugreek is a plant found in countries throughout southern Europe. It is cultivated in the central part of that continent and has become quite wild in fields, wooded slopes, and even among planted crops. The time for its flowering is in June and July.

Its medicinal uses are for inflamed throats, to reduce swellings and inflammation in wounds, and to prevent blood poisoning. It is used as a tea for reducing fevers.

Fenugreek is a plant which grows from six to eighteen inches high, and the leaves are triplicate, obovate leaflets. The flowers are single, double, or triple, and its seed pods are long, narrow, and sickle-like. The seeds are ground and are used as an ingredient of curry powder and for flavoring cattle food. They contain an alkaloid, trigonelline, and have been used medically. Fenugreek is grown for fodder in India, as it was in ancient Greece.

The *chicory,* or wild succory, is a plant which is native to Europe. It is now also cultivated in the United States. It flourishes in uncultivated places, by roadsides, on dry plains, and in dry ditches. It is a perennial herb.

Roasted and pulverized chicory roots are used in adulterating coffee or as a substitute for it. Tea prepared from the chicory roots has a purifying effect on the stomach, liver, spleen, and kidneys. Where there is an inflammation of the body, poultices of the whole plant may be applied to the parts affected. Alcohol in which the chicory root has been steeped is good as a rubbing lotion to remove weakness of the limbs.

Chicory is also said to be effective in jaundice, liver enlargement, gout, and rheumatic complaints, when made as a decoction of one ounce to one pint of boiling water.

When picked green, the leaves can be used as an appetizer and as a delicious salad or a vegetable, even during mid-winter.

9

Herbs and the Wheel
of the ECK-Vidya

Anyone who is a student of herbology and nutrition knows that in order to maintain or reestablish the normal equilibrium of the body, certain minerals must be present in proper proportions. A deficiency of any of the essential minerals in the body may result in functional disorders, including nervous exhaustion, with symptoms of mental and physical depression, anxiety, nervous dread, irritability, despondency, and brain fatigue, especially when intensified by overwork or worry.

One finds that in order to have perfect health in the world of matter, time, and space, where we live in the physical body and are subject to the laws of nature, one must learn to break agreements with his traditions, environment, and surroundings. One develops strength from the inner side of himself when he learns to make these shifts in himself.

This brings us to the *Bhavachakra,* the Wheel of Life, or that which those in Eckankar call the Cycle of the ECK-Vidya. The ECK-Vidya is a method of divination based upon the very ancient understanding of the Samsara, the world of changes. This is the Wheel of Life which is used by the Tibetans to inform the mind of man of the very nature of existence.

Within the ECK philosophy, it is found that one who has knowledge of this Wheel of Life is indeed fortunate. He knows there are twelve sections (representing the twelve months of the Western calendar) and that it takes twelve years to complete one cycle. This means that it takes 144 years to complete a full cycle of a single existence. This should actually be the length of every man's life on earth, but it is not, because of a lack of a proper balance of minerals in the body. As a result, few people live beyond the age of seventy-five.

Most ECK Masters will generally live to this age and beyond, according to the type of work they have to do while living here in their earthly bodies. Each ECK Master during his time here has constantly pointed out that each man is unique and that a set rule cannot apply to each individual, spiritually or physically.

Rebazar Tarzs, the great ECK Master, said, "Man has lived too long with the idea that there must be a single best way for him to do everything. He must change his traditional thinking of what is normal and average, so as to better understand the individual patterns in all aspects of his life. He must come to know himself."

The world is now a melting pot. Every country harbors a mixture of races. Each group has its own acquired habits, including nutritional habits. Orientals traditionally eat little meat, mostly because of its scarcity. But they get their protein from fish and soybeans. The Eskimos are largely meat eaters, because plant life in their world is scarce. Those living in the equatorial countries subsist primarily on plants and fruits.

We find that the size of portions, frequency of meals, and content of the meal varies considerably among people. Patterns are due to climate, habit, type of life, work, temperament, and physical body type. One's own heredity from his immediate family, his early childhood conditioning, and his emotional life patterns play an important part in the selection of foods.

The hunger for starches, sugar, and alcohol is a perverted appetite, according to Fubbi Quantz, who is the Abbot of the Katsupari Monastery in northern Tibet. People usually overeat carbohydrates, for they have no self-discipline concerning the appetite. Appealing only to the taste buds is certainly an incorrect approach to one of the most vital issues of physical and spiritual health.

The Wheel of the ECK-Vidya has twelve spokes, which are the original sections of time which have made up the calendar of all nations that have existed on earth. In ancient times there were thirty days in each month. This left five extra days, and the calendar would have to be adjusted periodically. In the course of time, however, the present calendar was worked out. In those ancient days the months were named for rare jewels.

We can somewhat compare the months of the present calendar with the ancient ECK calendar. They are as follows: January—the month of the emerald, called *Astik,* the days of wisdom; February—the month of the bloodstone, called *Uturat,* the days of love; March—the month of the jade, called *Garvata,* the days of joy; April—the month of the opal, called *Ebkia,* the days of hope; May—the month of the sapphire, called *Ralot,* the days of truth; June—the month of the moonstone, called *Sahak,* the days of music; July—the month of the ruby, called *Kamitoc,* the days of freedom; August—the month of the diamond, called *Mokshove,* the days of light; September—the month of the agate, called *Dzyani,* the days of friendship; October—the month of the jasper, called *Parinama,* the days of beauty; November—the month of the pearl, called *Hortar,* the days of wealth; and December—the month of the onyx, called *Niyamg,* the days of charity. According to the ancient knowledge handed down by the ECK Adepts, one should include in his daily diet certain foods during the varied months of the old calendar. This is based upon the vibrations of the physical and mental selves during these particular periods.

Health comes, of course, with the adjustment of the vibratory rates within one's self. This is what the ECK Masters do for anyone who approaches them for healing. The foods given here, which one should include in his diet for these varied months, should help in a similar way.

In *Astik* (January), the month of the emerald, one should have as much sage, valerian, lettuce, beans, nuts, and dried fruits included in his diet as possible.

In *Uturat* (February), the month of the bloodstone, one should have such foods as lettuce, seafood, green leafy vegetables, mushrooms, and mint in his diet.

In *Garvata* (March), the month of the jade, one should eat mainly watercress, onions, wheat germ, and chives. These will help balance inharmonies in the body.

In *Ebkia* (April), the month of the opal, one should include in his diet the following foods: apples, peppermint, almonds, grapefruit, figs, peaches, and spices.

In *Ralot* (May), the month of the sapphire, one should have in his daily meals caraway seed, cheese, seafoods, raisins, dates, peaches, apricots, and walnuts.

In *Sahak* (June), the month of the moonstone, one should have a certain limited amount of lean meats — mainly beef, chicken, turkey, and fish. Also included in the diet must be citrus fruits, tomatoes, raw cabbage, and seafoods which contain much iodine.

In *Kamitoc* (July), the month of the ruby, one should be very considerate of his diet by eating eggs, liver, saffron, cherries, oats, and fruits with pitted centers.

In *Mokshove* (August), month of the diamond, one should eat garlic, cheese, carrots, dried fruits, and lean meats. Pork should be excluded from the diet altogether.

In *Dzyani* (September), the month of the agate, one must include the following in his daily intake for better health: peaches, cherries, peas, and yellow vegetables. One should build up his energy and vitality as much as possible for the coming months of winter.

In *Parinama* (October), the month of the jasper, one should consume meat, eggs, fresh milk, dried fruits, and yellow vegetables. However, one must eat sparingly in order to give his stomach a rest from the past months of eating.

In *Hortar* (November), the month of the pearl, one must eat as much as possible of the following foods: asparagus, figs, carob, sage, cauliflower, turnips, turkey, chicken, and wild game, if it is available.

In *Niyamg* (December), the month of the onyx, one should consider in his diet fish, especially halibut and cod, whole grains, lean meats, baked potatoes, peas, corn, and beans.

The mineral chart, according to the old ECK calendar which corresponded with the months, is established as follows:

In *Astik* (January) we have the corresponding minerals which are best to be emphasized—phosphorus, bromine, and magnesium.

In *Uturat* (February) one should look to the following minerals in order to be healthier: iron, copper, and potassium.

In *Garvata* (March) one must look to the minerals which will make him a better thinker and give him good health around the upper part of his face and skull. These are fluorine, iodine, and sulfur.

In *Ebkia* (April) one should include in his daily nutritional intake, iodine, silicon, and fluorine.

In *Ralot* (May) one should think of the following minerals for better living—cobalt, silicon, and copper.

In *Sahak* (June) one should give more attention to potassium, sodium, and chlorine.

186

In *Kamitoc* (July) one must be very considerate of the minerals calcium, iodine, and chlorine.

In *Mokshove* (August) one should think carefully about adding to his daily diet foods which contain an abundance of sulfur, zinc, and the trace minerals.

In *Dzyani* (September) one must include in his diet the minerals sulfur, zinc, and cobalt.

In *Parinama* (October) one must consume those foods which will have a greater amount of magnesium, zinc, and copper.

In *Hortar* (November) one must look to phosphorus, calcium, and manganese for better health.

In *Niyamg* (December) nutrition for better health should include such minerals as phosphorus, sodium, and iron.

This is only a suggested chart, but it was used many centuries ago by the ancient peoples when ECK was a major faith and many followed it openly. Many of the minerals have already been discussed and will be further studied in later chapters, along with other important data about them.

Good health should be our birthright, but few have ever been this fortunate. In order to have greater relationships between one another and to give up the strain and stress of life, we must again take up the ancient ways of the ECK teachings. If we can come together as a world community again, as in the ancient, antediluvian days, the health of the individual will be more perfect.

The community life and ways the ancient ECK Masters planned for man to live are still possible today, if man will follow the perfect system. The most distinctive characteristic of such a social

187

organization, which includes a political and economic system, is a combination of autocratic rule and communal development. One-fourth of the agricultural crops and industrial products go to God to be placed in huge storeplaces for lean years; one-fourth go to the state; one-fourth go to the producers; and one-fourth go to the poor, aged, and infirm. Under such a system, poverty is rare and destitution is unknown. Society is organized as a collective one under a benevolent authority, who is usually the Mahanta, the Living ECK Master, or one who is appointed by him. Food is stored in special depositories as a defense against depression or lean years. An obligatory labor system is the basis of production and is self-serving. Social life is built around the family, not the individual. Clans are established in village communities. These communities have leaders who allot tasks, share rewards, and administer punishments.

The domains of religion, state, and community are merged in this social system. There is no profit system and no exchange of currency; labor is provided by cooperation. Ownership of land is communal, but families have their own homes which are private property. It is the socialist and free enterprise systems merged into one working modus operandi.

The world's people must find a system under which to live different than the present ones which are governing the various nations. This is not a criticism of any particular government, but of the social conditions existing throughout the world today.

Americans are considered the best fed, and, therefore, the healthiest people in the world. But this is not necessarily true. Few people, even in this country, have a knowledge of good nutrition, and nutrition is the key to good health and longevity.

Two-thirds of the world's population is underfed and suffers from infectious diseases. What we have failed to see in our antiseptic civilization is that disease and sickness develop an immunity to our artificial defenses. They seem to thrive even more on our constant fight to get rid of them than they do in those areas where sanitary conditions are more lax. A child who is raised in an environment without proper sanitary conditions will often develop a ruggedness which will give him an ingrained defense against disease and sickness. Whenever a person lives close to the soil and is able to get food from his garden, meat from the fields, and water from his well, he is getting more natural ingredients than those who live in cities.

As a nation, this country has an unusually large amount of sickness. It has been shown that at least nine hundred out of every thousand suffer from some defect and disorder. Statistics now show that one-third of the people during their life will be subject to cancer of one variety or another. The figures for those having heart trouble is supposedly thirty million. The latter is the number one killer in this country, due to the stress and strain of our modern civilization. Some twenty-seven million people are said to be arthritis victims. Diabetes patients run into a figure of about six million. Mental patients are said to make up another three million.

One wonders if nature, in some way, outwits our scientific and medical researchers in order to keep the population down. There are just as many children who die at an early age today, according to insurance company statistics, as there were before the advent of modern medicines. All this makes one ponder what the answer is for good health, longevity, and happiness.

As Science develops stronger antibiotics, the bacteria quickly become immmune to the new drugs, and stronger drugs are needed. The same applies to the other chemicals, such as pesticides, vermicides, nematocides, fungicides, and the whole gamut of insecticides that must be continually developed as the old standbys no longer do their job. We are quickly reaching the saturation point where the diseases and pests will have such a powerful immune system that man will have no defense against these perils.

Look at the yeast infection know as *Candida albicans*. It is no longer an epidemic but has now become pandemic. While almost everyone has some of this yeast in their bodies, one doctor now estimates that one third of the U.S. population may be adversely affected to some degree by *Candida*. It is a subtle disease that may not show any symptoms for a long time. But it can, and often does, end up being disastrous.

Yeast is everywhere. Fruits and vegetables are laced with yeast; the air is full of yeast; even mother's milk contains yeast. So it is impossible not to be subject to a yeast infection. We all are. Most people have a natural defense which keeps the yeast under control. According to some health authorities, this defense consists of a healthy culture of lactobacillus bacteria in the colon. The waste product of this bacteria is lactic acid, and it appears that this lactic acid production is one factor that keeps the normal yeast in the body at a controllable level.

The cholostrum produced by the mother during the first few days of nursing her newborn child contains immune globulins which carry antibodies to protect the child from infectious disease. The child is then provided with a normal supply of lactobacillus bacteria for protection. Within two weeks the mother will begin to produce normal milk without the protective antibodies, and the child's stomach will begin to produce hydrochloric acid; from then on it will be more difficult to restore the beneficial bacteria should they be destroyed.

Forty years ago, doctors advised mothers to use commercial baby formulas rather than breast feed their children. As a result, most of those children have little or no defense against yeast infection. About the same time, penicillin was introduced, and then hundreds of other antibiotics, which were used to treat a wide variety of illnesses. Often these drugs were true lifesavers, but more often they just destroyed the friendly bacteria in the colon — destroying the body's ability to ward off Candida.

So now we have set the stage for an outbreak of Candida. Many now consider Candida to be an iatogenic disease; one brought on by medicine or medical treatment. It also appears that our diet supports the growth of Candida. Diets high in sugar and carbohydrates seem to support the rapid growth of the yeast.

How does Candida harm us? It starts as a normal infestation of yeast that is controlled by the body's natural immunities. If the balance is upset by the destruction of the defending lactobacillus bacteria and a lowering of the body's immune system, there will be an explosive growth in the Candida population. It spreads throughout the body where it will inhabit the inner cell structure. Most infections live in the connective tissue outside the cells, where they break down the connective tissue (the collagen). When the connective tissue breaks down, it releases an active vitamin C which limits the infection somewhat. This doesn't happen with Candida, however, because of its tendency to inhabit the inner cell structure rather than living outside the cells.

As the Candida spreads, it is thought to produce a waste product, acetaldehyde, which also spreads through the body. This toxin can wreak havoc on the entire body, lowering the body's ability to produce energy from food, disrupting collagen production and fatty-acid oxidation. Being a potent blocker of the nerve synapses, acetaldehyde may also interfere with the nerve impulses to the various organs of the body. But the whole story of how Candida does its damage is not yet known.

Because it can permeate the entire body, the symptoms of Candida can mimic almost every other disease, and this makes diagnosis incredibly difficult. It can damage the kidneys, liver, heart, brain, eyes, muscles, and central nervous system. The results can be devastating. One researcher believes Candida may be connected to some cases of extreme allergies, autism, multiple sclerosis, schizophrenia, and toxic shock syndrome. Hopefully, soon we will have more answers than questions about Candida.

Few of us realize that it takes time to rebuild health and to discipline ourselves in the proper eating habits which will help take care of the body functions and structure.

We do not want to acquire a faddist attitude. Making food a fetish can also promote careless nutrition. Many believe they can have eternal youth by following certain dietary formulas, by the eating of particular foods, and by listening to those who promise nutritional cures for certain diseases. Hopefully, the intelligent person will readily identify those who are merely handing out propaganda and the scientific findings which soothe and lull millions into becoming complacent about their diets.

The United Nations conducted a survey through the World Health Organization to check the health of forty nations. The U.S.A. was fourteenth from the bottom (there were twenty-six nations in the world that had better health than the U.S.A. Only thirteen nations were sicker).

There has never been a large scale survey of the American diet which would lead anyone to the firm conclusion that we are well fed. Nor has there ever been a survey made of national health which would reveal that Americans are healthy people.

The practice of eating moderately of simple foods should be of vast importance to all. The habit of eating too much of even the best nutritional foods, or eating them in indigestible combinations with other foods, can be as bad as eating poor foods. It is true that we can live on about half of what we usually consume. Too many mothers will overfeed their children, mainly to satisfy their own natural desire to see them happier. Somehow or other, a child, in its native wisdom, manages to get enough to satisfy its vital needs. No child should be coaxed or urged to eat when not hungry. It is good to let him go without a meal once in a while if he does not appear to be hungry.

We find that the strict followers of religion, especially members of the Greek Orthodox church in southeast Europe, are known for their longevity. Their faith imposes dietary restrictions and frequent days of fasting. When the appetite is stimulated by great varieties of foods, we are usually tempted to eat far more than we should, because we wish to satisfy taste, rather than hunger.

Anyone can keep healthy on a small daily intake of food, provided the vitamins and minerals are sufficient. Any manual laborer or one who participates in sports can easily do well on a minimum of two meals daily, while the rest of us can make it on a single meal.

It is a well-known fact that if one tries to study or to seek spiritual enlightenment excessively, he will have a decrease of progress in this field. It is also known that if one gives a machine excess fuel, it decreases its power quite as readily as if it lacked fuel. The human body reacts in the same manner. If we overload the body with foods, it will soon stop functioning and begin to decay before its time. It often takes a long time before we can discipline the appetite, but if we do, then our weight will return to normal, and we can do our work more efficiently.

Since different types of food require different kinds of enzymes for digestive purposes, it is best to eat these foods separately. No one should combine concentrated proteins with concentrated starches (complex carbohydrates) in the same meal. When eating protein foods such as meats, fish, poultry, eggs, or cheese, it is best to combine them with green vegetables like lettuce, watercress, turnip greens, and celery.

Some health authorities will refute this idea, saying that certain natural foods contain both protein and starch. But when proteins and carbohydrates are consumed together, the carbohydrates will suppress the action of the protein-digesting enzymes, so the proteins will be only partially digested. However if no more than twenty percent of the food consists of high quality protein and the rest is unrefined carbohydrates, the enzymes will digest both proteins and carbohydrates.

It is a good nutritional practice not to eat large quantities of refined carbohydrates. In particular, do not combine complex carbohydrates (starches) with proteins. Your body will receive all the carbohydrates it requires from eating fruits, vegetables, and fish.

Proteins are the most difficult of foods to digest. To be used by the body, each protein chain must be broken down into shorter peptide chains, which are then broken down into amino acids before they can be used by the body. Soy protein is more difficult to digest than others because it has very long protein chains in its molecules.

It is best not to have more than one concentrated protein at a meal. For example do not combine meat with milk or eggs or fish and cheese. However, combining several ounces of one concentrated protein with four or five different proteins at a meal will assure that you are consuming all the necessary essential amino acids. For example, shrimp combined with alfalfa and sunflower sprouts and some sunflower and sesame seeds.

It is a good idea to have vegetables, some cooked, but mostly raw, with proteins. The vegetables will provide the enzymes that are so essential to the utilization of the proteins.

Whenever incomplete proteins are eaten, those which lack one or more of the essential amino acids, it is normal for the body to take the missing amino acid from its own tissues to complete the protein being digested. If the same kinds of protein are consistently consumed, a severe protein deficiency can develop as the body continues to make up the difference from its own supplies of amino acids.

It takes approximately six hours or longer for the body to process proteins, from the time you eat until the cells get the nourishment. If you can, eat these proteins early in the day to allow plenty of time for digestion before the body rests at night. When a protein meal is consumed late in the day and sleep comes before the body has had time to digest the protein, lymphatic congestion can occur. Should you experience digestive upset, gas, belching, indigestion, or related sleep disturbance, this is often the result of eating proteins too late in the day. Try eating the protein earlier in the day and without carbohydrates.

It is better not to snack on protein, as this will exhaust the digestive system. It would be better to have a snack of fruits, vegetables, and other unrefined carbohydrates.

On the other hand, do not mix acidic fruits with starches, as the acidity is bad for the enzymes upon which starch digestion depends. Such fruits as pine-apple, citrus, tomatoes, or any very sour fruit, will destroy the ptyalin enzyme upon which starch diges-tion is dependent. The first of the starch digestion is nullified, and the breaking up of the starchy intake then falls upon the pancreatic juices. One should drink any acidic juice, such as orange, grapefruit, or pineapple, at least fifteen minutes or more before eat-ing cereal. Those who obey this rule will generally eat acid foods or subacid foods alone.

It is best never to take two concentrated starches at the same meal. One should never combine bread and potatoes, as this leads to the overeating of a food that is required in small amounts only. This has nothing to do with the enzyme compatibilities, but such combi-nations lead only to overeating.

One must always remember that there is a limit to the effective functioning of the enzymes, and if one will provide the right food at each meal, then the digestive juices will function more efficiently.

If the body has its digestive functions impaired, the whole modus operandi will be out of regulation. The vital organs of the digestive tract, therefore, must be given deep thought and understanding, or one will suffer the consequences. This means that we cannot eat according to our likes and dislikes. Taste should not enter into the selection of foods at a meal.

The first consideration is to know what to drink. If fruits and vegetables make up a large proportion of our diet, then we do not require extra liquid. One should not have water at mealtimes, regardless of whether or not it is a fruit and vegetable meal. The habit of drinking water at a meal should not be encouraged, for it has the tendency to dilute the digestive fluids and flush vitamins and minerals from the body.

Chlorinated water or regular tap water is not good for the body health. Most tap water is no longer pure water, but a complex chemical solution which contains a number of additives, including fluorides.

As many as thirty-six different chemicals are regularly added to the tap water of our country. A partial list includes liquid chlorine, chlorine dioxide, copper sulphate, ammonia, sodium fluoride, lime, soda ash, carbon black, bone black, hydrochloric acid, polyelectrolytes, sodium chloride, and calcium chloride. Recent discoveries show that the chlorine in the water may combine with organic matter to produce chloroform which is a carcinogen (cancer producer).

Fluorine has been introduced into the public water system to reduce tooth decay in young children, but it has been found that over a period of years of drinking water which contains fluorine, damage to the kidneys, liver, and heart may result. We also find that chlorinated water uses up the vitamin E in the body, causing a loss of iodine.

The use of pure, natural spring water for body health, especially that which is bottled at the source, tends to increase vitality and maintain the vigor of those who use it. However, even natural spring water is no longer pure in many locations. Many health authorities now recommend the use of a quality water filter or distiller to remove any undesirable chemicals and pollutants from our water.

While on this subject, it has been pointed out that many synthetic fruit drinks and carbonated beverages are among the most unhealthy drinks available. Usually they consist of water colored with a coal tar dye, refined white sugar, corn syrup (glucose), with an added synthetic flavor, phosphoric acid, and caffeine. In all, they represent few vitamins and natural minerals for the body's intake. Virtually all soft drinks are sweetened with glucose — which many doctors believe is a prime cause of diabetes.

Only freshly squeezed juices contribute to good health. When one drinks these fresh juices, it will be found that his desire for synthetic and carbonated drinks will cease. The canned and bottled drinks have little, if any, enzymes. Processed drinks that are sold as reconstituted fresh juices are pasteurized and have preservatives to keep them appearing fresh to the consumer.

One may use coffee substitutes, such as cereal or dandelion coffees, which are available in practically every health food store. Too much regular coffee, as most health experts know, will create a deficiency of vitamin B, especially those elements of vitamin B called inositol and biotin. Enough caffeine will cause nervousness in the heavy consumer of coffee.

There are dozens of herb teas known for their respective healing power, such as chamomile tea for nervous troubles, mint tea for digestion, horehound tea for coughs and colds, and shave grass tea for the kidneys.

The trouble with regular tea is the caffeine and theobromine element, which is similar to caffeine in coffee. Theobromine destroys the nerve cells and

199

eventually interferes with the memory. Both tea and coffee lower the blood sugar. In those countries where tea is the main drink, people who are constant users will, over the centuries, become debilitated as a whole. As a group, their natural energies start going down. They become overwrought and highly emotional over very minute matters.

One of the greatest health hazards is refined white sugar. The disturbance of the body's calcium-phosphorus balance is brought about by an overuse of white sugar. The relationship of calcium to phosphorus is important in maintaining the proper proportion of minerals in the body.

By omitting white sugar and starchy diets there could be an elimination of dental cavities in our growing children. It is said that the Eskimos of Alaska had perfect teeth until modern civilization arrived in the north country. Today most of the Eskimos have false teeth before the age of twenty-five. This is due to the white sugar and dietary products made of refined foods which reached them through the coming of the white man into their world.

A better way to satisfy a sweet tooth without the use of products which contain refined, white sugar is a diet consisting of fruits, vegetables, whole grains, nuts, eggs, and milk. This provides the body with the equivalent of almost two cups of sugar daily. It also decreases the appetite for sweets. One particular point to make here is that sugar is not needed for energy, as we have been told by advertisers. Dried fruits contain about seventy-five percent carbohydrates, which are converted into sugar when digested. Anyone can nibble on dates, mission figs, and other dried fruits between meals in order to satisfy this type of hunger. Candies made from honey and carob are also useful as sweets. These can be found in most health food stores. Carob is often substituted for chocolate and sugar.

For good sources of natural sugars, well endowed with minerals and vitamins, one should try maple syrup and blackstrap molasses. Honey is another valuable, highly concentrated food, which gives vitality and general good health. It may also be used as a base in products for between-meal nibbling, especially for children.

Honey increases the hemoglobin count of the blood because of its content of copper, iron, and manganese. It is a quick way of getting energy, as it is largely predigested dextrose and does not have to go through the lengthy processes of body digestion. However, a little goes a long way.

Bananas are also a good source of energy and another way of satisfying the desire for sweets. When one eats a naturally ripened banana he gets calcium, phosphorus, iron, and vitamins A, B, and C. The average sized banana contains less than one hundred calories.

Egyptologists have found hieroglyphics of the pharaohs eating a gruel made of millet seed and dried figs. This was referred to as the Spirit-enlightening food of the pharaohs and was apparently used by them to increase their spiritual awareness.

Millet is the best whole grain for anyone, whether it is taken as hot breakfast food or made into a bread. It is high in protein, minerals, and vitamins and does not have the fattening effect of wheat.

Peasants throughout the Orient often must subsist on very small portions of food during time of famine. Many times they have gone through these starvation periods on a diet consisting mainly of millet. In some cases such diets have cured stomach ulcers and improved the health of those who have used them.

Rice is not the universal food in Asia, except in the south. The northern areas grow millet as the staple food and have done so since recorded time. We will find that the population is stronger and more vigorous in the north than in the other areas where the populace lives entirely on rice as the staple food.

There are four foods which will help one maintain the standard needs of vitamins and minerals in the body. They are kelp, which furnishes practically every mineral needed by the body; citrus fruits, for vitamin C; brewer's yeast, which gives B-complex vitamins; and wheat germ oil, which contains vitamin E. With the B-complex and vitamin E added to one's daily intake of food, he should have exceedingly good health.

10

The Sacred Herbs of the ECK Masters for Longevity

For centuries, the principal food of the poor has been bread, and bread is still the chief ingredient of the diets of many poor people in remote areas of the world. One cannot live on carbohydrates, starches, and sugar without suffering from the effects of this type of eating.

It can be noted without having to resort to statistics that the death rate among the poorest of people is high compared to that of those who are able to furnish themselves with better nutrition. The Industrial Revolution brought with it the need for cheap, nonperishable foods for urban areas, where man had to congregate in order to make a living in industry and where he was not in a position to raise his own food.

Because of this, the methods of processing foods were developed. Unfortunately, processing removed many of the life-giving nutrients, leaving nothing but starches. What was taken out went to feed animals, so that they would be in good health to serve as dairy animals or to be slaughtered and fed to the people of the cities.

The present young generation is not as bright and intelligent as we believe. The British have collected results of tests given English school children, age eleven, since 1914. According to Sir Cyril Burt, in spite of the vast improvement made in social conditions during the last fifty years and the alleged improvements in educational methods, there have been no signs whatever that the average level of intelligence has been raised. Nor has there been any discernible leveling of the intelligence of the duller children, nor any indication that the proportion of brighter children has grown.

Of course, there have been fads in reading methods, spelling, and other facets of education. The advent of television has brought about a certain amount of learning, but this is not intelligence. Learning is the art of logical self-expression and the ability to draw conclusions from experiences.

We find that fifty to one hundred years ago parents were in a much better position to put on the table food which was fresh from the soil or unprocessed. This may be the reason why we have had such a leveling of intelligence. Vitamins, minerals, and other life-sustaining factors are withdrawn from processed foods and substitutes often replace them. As a result, the daily diet today has become fifty percent concentrated starch and sugar, practically all of which has been deprived of the elements needed to sustain life.

Poor health created by too much sugar and starch has caused many people to take drastic measures for healing. Often one can be the victim of advertising, tradition, or plain ignorance, because the general public has never been educated in good nutrition. We also have religious influences which regulate the diet of millions. Many people would starve rather than eat bacon and eggs for breakfast. Others would never touch meat from a cow.

Also, we have to consider the ethnic aspects of nutrition. Ethnic influences have created more problems for people than religious biases. We also have the faddists and cultists who are willing to listen to anyone who can make even a vague promise to rid one from defects and illnesses through nutrition.

Most people do not realize that the stress of hard work can cause a depletion of such critical vitamins as C, B_1, and the readily utilizable fatty acids of the polyunsaturated types. There may also be critical shortages of magnesium, potassium, and calcium. Most hard working people seem to have a major deficiency in fresh, natural, unheated oils from grains, such as wheat germ oil. This could be, according to health authorities, because they tend to eat a heavy carbohydrate diet and neglect other foods, especially green, yellow, and red vegetables and fresh fruits.

No longer do we eat food grown in the soil where we live that contains the minerals of which our bodies are made. Most of our ancestors were born and lived in the same community. The minerals in the soil and water become a part of the individual.

Some believe that foods grown at a particular longitude and latitude will have certain magnetic characteristics that are unique for that location and that these characteristics will also appear in a person

205

living in that area. Thus, it is felt that locally-grown food will be more beneficial to a person than food grown in an entirely different area.

Foods should be grown as close to where one lives as possible and should be eaten as soon after being harvested as possible. The commercialization of food may be one of the biggest problems facing man. Anything which is done to food from the time it is mature or harvested, destroys some of its vitality, and this includes storage, freezing, processing, or transporting it to farflung distribution points.

Our ancestors had longevity, and few of us do today because we are eating potatoes grown in Maine or Idaho, eggs from chickens raised in the deep South, meat that comes from the West, grain that is raised in the Midwest, and vegetables from California and Florida. So little food comes from the soil where we are living. Our longevity has taken a drop, and we are unable to find what is wrong with ourselves when we reach the end of our body's endurance because of a lack of minerals and vitamins.

Most Americans would die on the diet regimen of the Orientals, because their bodies have become used to a different diet. The city restaurants of Akita, Japan, serve what is considered to be the secret of a long and vigorous life. Akita is a city on the Omono River near the Sea of Japan, on northern Honshu, and is noted for its main meal called *shottsuru ryori*.

The special dish in this meal is similar to *sukiyaki*. The difference is that chunks of carp fish are used instead of beef, and the liquid in which all is simmered is the elixir which is said to give long life and which is found only at Akita.

206

In other places the liquid used is the usual type made with a fish base. But in Akita the elixir of life is said to be that of an ancient recipe. It is made of hormones which have been buried underground for a considerable length of time so that they may ripen like wine. The restaurant owners put considerable stock in their recipe of the shottsuru ryori because the women remain younger and more beautiful than in other cities and the men more youthful and vigorous. It seems that perhaps they have discovered something that the rest of the world knows little about.

Many accept the idea that death between the ages of sixty-five and seventy is normal, although science says that death at such an age is premature and could be due to undernourishment of the cells of the body. One thought is that old age is due to the diminished capacity of the organs which make the cells of the body. They can no longer function in the reproduction of cells that make up the body tissues. Those tissue cells are important; if they have the necessary nutrition, they will promptly remove all wastes and poisons from the body and function for an extended length of time, increasing the span of the body's life. If this is true, then the answer to long life lies in finding the proper herbal remedies to nourish the tissues. Our ancestors knew the properties of the beneficial herbs and roots that grew in the woods and fields, which are gradually regaining their place in modern medicine.

One of the most important herbs, and one known to the ECK Masters for centuries, is the *fo-ti-tieng*, or *Hydrocotyle asiatica minor*, a plant with extraordinary rejuvenating effects on the human brain cells and endocrine glands. Some scientific and medical researchers say it contains an unknown vitamin. Since this vitamin has not been fully researched, it has been given the name of vitamin X.

The herb is found only in the marshy, jungle areas of Ceylon, south China, and southwest Asia. With ginseng, which has already been discussed elsewhere in this book, gotu kola, and sarsaparilla, this ancient, but recently rediscovered, plant has given man hope for longevity.

There is considerable confusion about fo-ti-tieng today. One product is available called Fo-Ti-Tieng, which is a registered trademark. It is a combination of three herbs. There is also an herb which is sold as fo-ti-tieng or fo-ti which is listed as *Polygonum multiflorum*. In China, this herb is known as ho shou wu.

Fo-ti-tieng is called the "Elixir of Life" or "Long Life Elixir." It is not a plant which would attract the attention of most people, yet it has become well known among Chinese and Indian scholars as a food which contains a great life-sustaining property. Its action is aromatic, corrective, diuretic, and nutritive. It is also used as a stimulant and a tonic. It has several uses as a remedy besides being a defense against old age. It is used to combat fevers, piles, bowel complaints, and scrofulous conditions. It is said to strengthen and energize the brain. A few leaves a day are taken, but it appears that they are chewed, rather than drunk in a tea.

The plant grows only a few inches high and is a rather dull green color. The leaves are green and fan-shaped. The roots appear to be extremely long, perhaps twice the length of the plant stem above ground.

Of course, at this length, the roots would be able to absorb the minerals of the soil in which it grows. This plant always grows in remote marshy areas.

Fo-ti-tieng does possess the virtue of promoting good health and longevity. It is not necessary to eliminate meat or flesh proteins, as so many do for the sake of gaining long life; the leaves of the fo-ti-tieng may be ground up and put in with stews and soups. It is said to produce a general sense of good feeling, clear thinking, energy, and an improvement in appearance.

Many of the ECK Masters during the early days on this planet developed the fo-ti-tieng for the purpose of helping people overcome many of their ailments and create a good life without pain and unhappiness. However, in the past few centuries, the practice has died out because they have found that it brought about more of an interest in the material side of life rather than the spiritual.

The ECK Masters have specific spiritual exercises which give them longevity. These extraordinary Adepts of the East are actually God-eaters, not in the symbolic sense that the Christians eat the body of Christ in the sacramental host and drink the Savior's blood as wine, but the ECK Masters eat the cosmic energy which is the ECK, that spiritual power which flows out of God. They do this purposely for survival, the same as man eats material food to keep his body alive.

Until one learns to live outside the physical state of consciousness in the Soul body, he cannot hope to progress to such a spiritual life as the God-eaters, the *Eshwar Khanewale*. The God-eaters live in a strange city called Agam Des, one of the spiritual cities of the world located near the tremendous peak of Tirich Mir in central Asia, which rises to the height of 25,230 feet. It is the highest point in the Hindu Kush range of mountains which border Kashmir, Afghanistan, and Pakistan.

Agam Des means the inaccessible world, and it certainly is, for not only is its position hidden deeply in these remote wilds, but no one is allowed there unless by invitation from the ancient brotherhood of the God-eaters. When one goes there, it must be done by the *Nuri Sarup,* the Light body, escorted by the Living ECK Master.

When one first hears of this mysterious group of Adepts and their incredible teachings, he finds it all very hard to believe. They are said to be in control of the secret forces of the cosmic life which gives human history its many changes and shapes in this world.

It was only after I had made contact with the great ECK Master, Rebazar Tarzs, that I became acquainted with the Eshwar Khanewale in their secret city of Agam Des. Tarzs also brought to my attention the deeper knowledge of Eckankar, the Ancient Science of Soul Travel. The basic credo of the spiritual works of ECK is that man is a spiritual Co-worker with God, that man has access to liberation and freedom in this lifetime, and that he always has existed, and always will exist throughout eternity as Soul.

It is through supernatural energy that the God-eaters can supervise the spiritual law. They have this ability because the supernatural energy is secondary to the knowledge of the spiritual law.

When one learns to live in the other worlds, he is then able to give up the foods of this earth world and live as the God-eaters, who consume the ECK as their food. St. Catherine of Siena was an eater of the Cosmic Spirit, as is Rebazar Tarzs, the great ECK Master who has lived here since 1452. Other great ECK Masters who are adepts in the art of survival through Spirit are: Fubbi Quantz, head of the Katsupari Monastery in the northern Tibetan mountains, who is several centuries older than Rebazar Tarzs; Sudar Singh, my first ECK Master in India, who was 105 years old at the time of his death; the old Chinese ECK Master, Suto T'sing, who lived for 267 years in the same body; the well-known Chinese ECK Master, Lai Tsi, who is the head of the Temple of Golden Wisdom located in the Etheric world, who lived on earth for a half dozen centuries. Heading up the order of the ECK Masters is Yaubl Sacabi, whose age is beyond human conception. He is the head of the city of Agam Des, and a leading ECK Master of the Order of the Vairagi here in this world.

The ancients learned the extension of consciousness and moved into the higher states, proving that longevity is possible. The art of good health comes with the knowledge and ability of Soul Travel. We find that Soul Travel can be used for self-healing and will take us into the world of good health and prosperity. But not many of us will become like the Adepts of Eckankar, many of whose bodies last for centuries, because we have no purpose for living this long in this world.

These God-eaters absorb the ECK, the cosmic energy, at a fantastic rate. By doing so, they use their physical bodies to serve the planets, including the earth world, and the inner planes which are the Astral, Causal, Mental, Etheric (subconscious), the Atma (Soul), and the planes of pure Spirit. They serve, not merely because the spiritual law demands service to all beings, but also in self-interest, for should the atmosphere become too loaded with radiation they will move to another planet or higher universe. They work best from the earth planet, because the flow of cosmic particles is greater here than in the other parts of this physical universe.

The reason we wear this physical body for a few score years is due to our karmic debt. Unless we dispose of this karmic debt we must go from one lifetime to another in various incarnations. The only way that one can become free of this karmic debt in a relatively short time is by finding the Living ECK Master, and eventually being initiated by him. This initiation takes one off the Wheel of the Eighty-Four, which is that treadmill of rebirth and death in this physical universe.

There is another method of rejuvenating body health known as the *Ayur Vedha,* a system of renewing the health and youth of the physical body. One offshoot of the Ayur Vedha is known as the *Kaya Kalp,* which means life-time. In other words, it offers a second life. Kaya Kalp is part of a system of spiritual practices which is somewhat known in India, but only a few of the ashrams in the Orient give it as part of their rejuvenation practice. One of these ashrams is in south India, another in the Himalaya mountains, one in the Katsupari Monastery in the remote northern Tibetan mountains, and one in western China.

The concepts of rejuvenation are based upon the unique idea that in the body of man (which is a living and functioning organism, independent of the mind, yet influenced by it) is a spiritual energy and a Kal (negative) energy. These energies are generally kept at a balance during the time of a person's life on earth. But as one grows older, the Kal energies take over a little at a time until the balance is all in its favor; then death occurs.

It is for this reason that man grows old. If his work or the pressures of his daily life are great, this overbalance can come before his normal span of life is finished for this incarnation. If he does not have proper nutrition, a proper attitude toward life, or a proper knowledge about life, this balance can grow more rapidly on the negative side, bringing him to physical death more quickly.

The idea of the Kaya Kalp is to increase the span of life by raising the ECK forces in the human body so that the balance will be brought in favor of the positive side of the energies.

The Kaya Kalp cure consists of a dieting program in which the only foods eaten are taken directly from the soil and prepared especially for the particular person whose body system is lacking in certain minerals and vitamins. Among these foods are the famous herbs which are known for the restoring of the vital energies of the body.

First is the Asiatic ginseng which is called "The Man Plant" by the Chinese. They have used it for over five thousand years as a health tonic and to prolong human life. It is said to help the sick recover, to make the healthy stronger, and to reactivate the entire human organism.

213

Although this herb has been discussed in another chapter, it is well to point out here that today in China and India men over fifty include it regularly in their diet in order to preserve their virility.

Another rejuvenation herb used in the same system of Kaya Kalp is *gotu kola.* It is said that a few leaves eaten raw daily will strengthen and revitalize the body and brain. It is supposed to be the essential factor in the extreme age reached by elephants in Ceylon where the herb grows wild.

Gotu kola has pale green, fan-shaped leaves and is a ground creeper. When mixed with regular food and served daily in the diet of anyone, health is restored and one is able to live to a ripe old age. It is grown in India, the islands of the Indian Ocean, and some parts of South Africa. The natives of India use the plant medicinally as a diuretic to stimulate the kidneys and bladder.

Fo-ti-tieng is vastly important in the Kaya Kalp. Its properties exert a rejuvenating influence on the ductless glands, the healthy functioning of which keeps the brain and body in good health.

Sarsaparilla is used in a limited way. The root, according to reports, contains hormones and is beneficial in bringing about vitality in a person who has lost his ability to produce children because of disease, accident, or old age.

It is said that three types of hormones are found in the sarsaparilla root. These are the hormones testosterone, progesterone, and cortin. Various experiments have shown that the administration of the male hormone, testosterone, tends to restore the vitality and to bring about mental alertness and physical

214

strength to men who are entering the stage of physical decline. In a sense this hormone prolongs youth and prevents premature aging.

If we want to keep well and have a long life, then it is wise to see what those in charge of the Kaya Kalp program do with the diets of their people. They provide the following minerals for those participating in the Kaya Kalp:

Lime or calcium salts are found in every tissue. They are particularly essential to the teeth, bones, nails, hair, and muscle development. They improve the stamina, are beneficial to the nerves, and help the pulse.

Phosphorus is likewise essential to the bones, teeth, supple tissues, and to stimulate growth. It is also present in the cell nuclei and vital to the brain. The body needs phosphorus in a ratio of four units of phosphorus to every ten units of calcium. Too much calcium and the body becomes alkaline; too much phosphorus and the body tends to be acid.

Iron is vital to the blood. It forms the red pigment, hemoglobin, and assists in the carrying of oxygen from the lungs to the tissues. It also is of importance to metabolism and helps anemia, sallow complexion, poor appetite, and adrenal gland trouble arising from a lack of iron salts in the blood.

Iodine is a food mineral which has been found to be deficient in the modern diet of man. It is essential to the thyroid gland which controls the metabolism of the body and our emotional reactions. Iodine foods prevent goiter, strengthen the nerves, are beneficial in kidney disorders and in adjusting the physique to better proportions when either too fat or too thin.

215

Manganese plays a part in the process of reproduction and growth. It is also important for the brain and nerves.

Other minerals which help prolong the body's life are potassium and magnesium. They are both essential because of their part in body health, which is similar to the function of calcium salts.

Copper is usually associated with iron in food substances and is essential to its assimilation by the body.

Other items which the Kaya Kalp treatment takes up are: physical exercises coordinated to supply blood to every part of the body, special massages, and relaxation exercises for mind and body.

There is abstinence from social activity while undergoing the treatments. In special mental concentration exercises, one learns to develop a calm mental attitude and to clear the mind of all worldly thoughts. Poisonous elements such as worry, temper, and passion are erased from the mind. A determination and will to live longer is developed which is close to self-hypnosis.

The results of the Kaya Kalp depend upon the individual. A complete treatment may take a few months or a year. As a result the positive energy is increased, decaying tissues are removed and replaced with the youthfulness and strength of new body energies. The determination to live longer is now a natural part of the character.

Anyone who is able to find and take treatments of the Kaya Kalp should increase his life span at least twenty to thirty years. It is found that the health and vigor of one's youthful years will return, gray hair disappear, and he will be able to sire children again.

However, one cannot expect to find the places where these treatments are given unless he is willing to serve humanity in some manner. Not everyone is able to take such treatments of the Kaya Kalp system, because if this were so, the world might be flooded with all sorts of persons who have longevity, but who take advantage of it by gaining control of communities, states, and nations for their own advantage. The fortunate ones are carefully selected by those in charge.

The same holds true of anyone who is able to visit the spiritual city of Agam Des. The only people who can do this are those who have been selected by the ECK Masters to make such trips by Soul Travel. Yaubl Sacabi, the ancient ECK Master in charge of this strange city, does not allow just anyone there— even those who might wander upon it by chance. He is probably the oldest of any being who lives on this planet, but he appears to be a man in his late thirties. Occasionally, those who participate in the works of ECK can reach the spiritual city of Agam Des. But again, it is only via the invitation of the ECK Masters that one can reach it and enjoy the works of these strange adepts.

H3, which is a factor in procaine hydrochloride, has been used frequently by authorities to help older people regain health and to expand life. It is said that procaine HCl is non-habit forming, well tolerated in the body, and above all, not a narcotic. It can be bought openly without a prescription.

H3 was developed in Rumania under government supervision and was first used with older people for treatment of the signs of age. Early experiments were deemed successful, and research has been done in many countries and has progressed into what is known as Gerovital H3 therapy. It is said that the experiments here in this country have been successful, and some value was found in treating hypertension, irregular heart rhythm, angina pectoris, skin inflammation, hives, and narcotics addiction.

H3 seems to have been successful in helping the elderly restore memory, energy, hearing, dulled mental faculties, and in treating rheumatism, diseases of the cardiovascular system and the gastrointestinal system. Apparently, H3 will be further developed, and some announcement will be made in the future as to the results of experiments by medical research teams.

Longevity normally belongs in the area of family characteristics. While some families are noted for their long span of life, some are notoriously short-lived. Those living in rural areas where life is slower, tempers are more even, and there is less chance of eating foods which have been processed, are apt to have a greater life span than their city cousins. This has been found to be true in Hunza, where a number of people are advanced in age, but appear to be middle-aged or younger. Some persons claiming to be over 110 years of age are cropping up in remote corners of the world. Lately such reports have been received from the deep rural areas of Russia, as well as Turkey and the Baltic countries.

There are several reasons for this. First, is family stock. If the family stock is strong, tough, and healthy, the body does not weaken and succumb to disease like those who are living under strain and stress

218

in the metropolitan areas. Second, many are living in such deep rural sections of the country that they have to live directly off the land, and the soil of these lands could possibly contain minerals and vitamins which are important to the body. Since food is not so plentiful where people have to raise and cultivate their own food products, it is possible that they do not have so much to eat as in other places. Too often the body is overfed and this creates a problem, for it is more easily weakened and can fall victim to disease and illness. It is best to skimp on food rather than overeat.

Another reason may be that people living in these areas can find plants such as ginseng, fo-ti-tieng, and gotu kola to supplement their nutritional needs. This would, of course, establish greater longevity, and they would naturally retain youth, vitality, and those factors which give the body long life when others are struggling to keep free from sickness and health problems.

In the onrush of civilization, man acquired the idea that he must accumulate possessions by pushing ahead and driving himself into a frenzy. In the process of this he has lost the inner ability to replenish that spiritual self which is the sustainer. Consequently, he has undergone great strain which wears out his bodily strength and resistance. The foods with which he feeds his body lack nourishment, and he has no time to rest, to be silent, to try his spiritual exercises, and to relax. Nervous tension sets in and shortens his life. No man who is easily irritated can have complete peace of mind, because his nerves, muscles, and brain are constantly under great tension.

Therefore, he seeks out healers who work by spirit. This is good, but he must give full consideration to what he is doing. There must be practical sense applied to his finding the right healer who is going to give him back his health, if this is possible. It is the same yardstick by which he would find the right healer in the physical medicine field.

The idealist is drawn toward the mystical and transcendental by his desire to lift the burden of suffering from humanity. He is aware of the limitations of orthodox methods, and he hopes to escape from these limitations. While he does not condemn spiritual healing, he must look very deeply into the whole subject. He cannot shut his eyes to the unsatisfactory and disastrous results that happen when spiritual healing has been ignorantly or inadequately employed.

Good intentions are no substitute for sound knowledge. The satisfactory healer is one who has an adequate knowledge of the physical, psychic, mental, and spiritual nature of man. He must know how they correlate with one another. They fit together like the layers of skin on the body, each essential function in its place.

Even the most extreme spiritual healers do not expect any man to grow a new arm or leg. The greatest mistake that healers make is failing to recognize that each plane has its own laws. They must recognize where the problem lies and work from this plane to help nature take its course.

Other factors, too, enter into healing, such as the karmic pattern of other lives which may influence the present life and must be worked out. When the Living ECK Master recognizes this in his chela, he

220

stands aside and allows the karma to work itself out. He can also recognize when one is suffering from strain because of the pressures in his life, or when a lack of proper vitamins, minerals, and nutritious foods have brought the chela to the edge of a nervous breakdown. Also, he knows there is a time and place for spiritual healing, as well as a time and place for medical treatment. He never interferes with the latter, for medicine has its place.

Spiritual healing has its limitations whether the healer admits it or not. He cannot blatantly tell the victim of some physical, psychic, or spiritual problem that, "you are healed," and walk away. He must also consider the spiritual level of the person who approaches him. If he who requests healing has a low survival factor, he is not apt to be healed spiritually.

If he has a chronic negative attitude, it is not likely that anyone can do much for him. However, if he has a positive, cheerful attitude, it is most likely that he can have a healing, which can often be called a miracle.

No healer in his right mind would make a diagnosis of anyone's problems and prescribe, unless it is on a spiritual level. The healer is limited in his work, and if he believes that he has the power to cure anyone who has the breath of life in him, he is apt to be heading straight into trouble. He cannot diagnose and prescribe, because he has not had the background nor the training to do so. He is being naive if he believes that he can heal anyone who comes to him. He must not make rash promises that he can heal anyone who approaches him with a problem.

Nor should he accept anyone who comes to him in regard to relatives, friends, or family members to be healed. Anyone who wants healing should approach the healer personally. The same principle applies here that applies in the physician's office. Nobody goes to the doctor and asks that he treat an absentee patient.

Most people approach the spiritual healer for two reasons. First, they are naive and believe that they can be healed. This is not faith but sort of a traditional belief that God takes care of anyone who asks. Second, many people are afraid to see their physicians and learn the truth about themselves. A certain percentage want the service of healing without paying or rendering full price for it. Yet they will pay in some way, for this is the way life works.

11

Health Secrets of the ECK Adepts

Those who live the longest and have the most enjoyment of life seem to have a greater amount of intelligence and are more vital in their love, work, and family life than others. For some reason they appear to be wealthier as well.

Married people have longer lives than single, divorced, or widowed people. The active sex life in a marriage appears to give one a stronger survival in the physical body and, of course, animation and vitality. Those who smoke and drink in moderation are going to have a longer life expectancy than those who do so in excess. Those who do not smoke and drink at all will have a far better survival for longevity in the physical body.

Good health is naturally one of the dividends earned as a result of good nutrition and wholesome living from birth to the present time. Good diet will always prolong youth, and whether one is going to have serious illnesses in his twenties, thirties, or fifties depends in large measure upon the choice of food given him from the formative years to his present decade. It can be said that the characteristics of senility may not be the mark of old age, but rather of poor nutrition.

Good nutrition slows the aging process, while poor nutrition accelerates the processes of physiological and psychological aging. Malnutrition can rapidly bring about the appearance of old age. The hair loses its color, the skin wrinkles, and the vital organs develop malfunctions while chemical changes of the body come about.

Magnesium is required for good mentality. It is often called the mineral of life because it is very vital to the core of all the physical makeup of the body. The motor nerves are dependent on magnesium to conduct the electrical impulses from the brain to the muscles. Magnesium makes the difference in the performance of the motor nerves, whether it is going to be slow and labored, or quick, smooth, and well-coordinated.

Magnesium also helps to maintain normal blood pressure and to build strong bones and teeth. Magnesium dissolves and prevents kidney stones, speeds healing, and helps lower serum cholesterol. Magnesium is the mineral for keeping the memory in good working order. A new pill has been developed called the "memory pill" which has magnesium as its base.

Magnesium also regulates the functions of cells other than bones. It gives energy to the vital part of the normal cells because of the oxidation of glucose through the enzymes. The process which activates the enzymes requires magnesium.

This releases a whole chain of action. The enzymes activated by magnesium mediate the movement of muscles, the process of breathing, storage of energy, digestion of food, building of tissues, reproduction, workings of the brain, and even the thought processes; all are the results of the activating force of this particular mineral.

If anyone is living in a metropolitan area where the water has been artificially fluoridated, more magnesium intake is needed. The best source of magnesium is dolomite, nuts, sunflower, and pumpkin seeds.

Vitamin E is a stopgap for the aging process in the body. It prevents oxygen from combining with the essential fatty acids to form peroxides and free radicals. The latter cause the cells to die and impede the action of the important enzymes. The body energy lessens, and the body's ability to renew itself is diminished. One begins to age in body and face.

Should the consumption of fats outbalance the amount of vitamin E available, we have another youthful vitamin, *vitamin C,* stepping in. Vitamin C works like a cleanser, sweeping up the troublesome free radicals which are formed from too much fat consumption, breaking them down, and eliminating them through the body's natural elimination system. This is why one needs more vitamin C as he grows older.

Vitamin C joins forces with vitamin E to help in the prevention of the peroxides. But there must always be enough vitamin C in the daily diet or in supplements to be effective on two lines of battle against old age. It plays both an offensive and defensive role for the body's health.

225

Another way to a happy old age is that of the *nucleic acids*. These are the building blocks of life and are an essential part of the genetic process and participate in the renewal of the body cells. Some of the nucleic acids form the DNA which controls heredity and the subsequent ability of the body to keep reproducing its inherited patterns of life.

This DNA can carry the genetic code for a longer life free of degenerative disease with the quality of feeling young as long as the individual lives.

The pharaohs of ancient Egypt formed a closed shop on outsiders, marrying their own sisters and cousins to keep the throne intact. But the genetic defects of the family kept reproducing in subsequent generations. Therefore, the successors to the throne were usually the children of the non-royal wives.

One of the greatest of the pharaohs was Thutmose II, who expanded his empire beyond the boundaries of those kings before him. Like his father, he was an illegitimate child. The most famous of the pharaohs was Amenhotep IV, the son of a Nubian mother who was a court woman without any rank of royalty. He is known to us as the first pharaoh who tried to establish a single god. He also founded a new capital and new laws. In tradition he married his mother, his cousin (the famous Egyptian beauty, Nefertiti), and his daughter. But Tutankhamen, the second son-in-law to succeed him and the only surviving male heir to the throne, was the child of a non-royalist wife. Marriages to close relatives did not produce longevity, for the nucleic acids in DNA and RNA, which should renew themselves and keep their patterns of genetic information as clear and distinct as possible, cannot do so in interfamily marriages.

Brewer's yeast is said to be one product rich in nucleic acids. Besides yeast, other foods which are rich in these acids are seafoods of all kinds, especially small sardines and herring roe. Organ meats, particularly sweetbreads, help to stop aging in man.

It is interesting to note the ages of some of the Greeks of ancient times. Sophocles composed his magnificent *Oedipus at Colonus* at age ninety. Agesilaus II, king of Sparta, died at eighty-four while commanding Spartan mercenaries. Socrates changed the current of human thought without writing a word, without preaching a doctrine, simply by talking in the streets of Athens, which he left but twice in defense of the city. At seventy-one, he was still vigorously defending his philosphies when he was sentenced to death and drank the poison hemlock. Aeschylus was sixty-nine when he died, and he had already written his own epitaph. Euripides died at seventy-eight and was composing plays till he died; his last, *Alcmaeon of Corinth,* won a posthumous prize in Athens. Protagoras died in a shipwreck at seventy-five, while Aristophanes lived till he was sixty-five. Plato died at eighty; Isocrates at ninety-eight. Gorgias died at 107. And this was during a time when historians believe that the average lifespan was about twenty years.

One begins to wonder about the longevity of these famous Greeks and any possible connection with their diet and the soil their food was grown in. It seems that the Greeks of that time lived mostly on bread, a few olives, barley meal, a little wine, and fish. And yet this diet seems to have bred a vigorous race of men.

It is possible that the ancient Greeks received the right minerals, vitamins, and nucleic acids from fish, and the necessary vitamin E from fish and whole grains. Their bread was made directly from wheat gathered in fields without any processing other than grinding into flour. Grapes furnished a source of vitamin C. Seeds and berries also likely furnished the rest of what was needed for the body's supply of vitamin C for longevity.

One traditional medicine, called *Kampō,* is still relied upon in Japan. It originated in the tradition of Chinese medicine, which prescribes concoctions prepared from plants, leaves, grass, and roots.

Kampō is entirely different from modern medicine, especially from the standpoint of diagnostics or its conception of the human body. Modern medicine is based on scientific analysis, while Kampō depends upon the practitioner's intuition and observation.

The physician in Kampō tries to grasp the condition of the patient in a whole view. It is the nature of the Eastern philosopher to adapt himself to the whole instead of to the parts. This is the way he is trained from childhood. Whatever he would prescribe for the patient would be prepared from grass, leaves, tree trunks, bark, roots, and herbs. These are all natural products, but the portions vary according to the complaint.

Until modern medicines were introduced into Japan, only the technique of Kampō was used. It has suffered somewhat the same results as many elements of Japanese culture and has been partly forgotten by some of the newer generations. But in the past few years it has become popular again, for many people of Japan are seeking out Kampō practitioners.

The Kampō physician inspects the patient using his own intuition and feelings. He is generally one who has had many years of experience, as well as a sharp medical intuition.

The examination includes four separate points. These are: questions, visual examination, tactual examination, and smell. The Kampō physician accepts everything the patient says as part of the examination. His whole analysis is based upon the subjectiveness of what is learned beyond the objective or scientific examination given by the Western physician. The Kampō doctor listens to the patient, obtains information about his family, his medical history, living conditions, environment, and anything which can add to the knowledge needed for diagnosis. At the same time, he is giving the patient a physical checkup.

When the examination is finished, he determines the proper treatment. The physician is looking for a pattern of symptoms known as the *shō*, which is the concept unique to Kampō. It is not found in Western medicines.

The materials which compose Kampō prescriptions are natural grasses, plants, and their components, although some are of animal and mineral origin. The effective ingredients are contained in living medicines, which can be naturally assimilated by the human body. A single formula may contain ten ingredients, and there are as many as twenty formulas for the common cold, depending on the symptoms. While chemical medicines can cause allergies or irritations, Kampō does not do this, according to claims, nor does it put a burden on the digestive and assimilative organs.

Kampō had its origin in the western part of China, south of the Yangtze River. The climatic conditions provided for the natural growth of roots, barks, grasses, and herbs, which were discovered useful to the body some two thousand years ago.

The Chinese book which described the medical treatment upon which Kampō is based was the *Shang han za bing lun* (*Essay on Typhoid and Miscellaneous Diseases*, typhoid referring to all fevers). This was written by Zhang Ji in about 150 A.D. Later, in about 1000–1300 A.D., it was divided into two parts, the *Shang han lun* (*Essay on Typhoid*) and the *Jin kui yao luë* (*Synopsis of the Golden Chamber*). The Kampō physician will use these as a reference for the prescriptions; these books include the essentials of the modern system of Kampō. It was not until about the sixth and seventh centuries that such treatments were able to reach Japan. Japan accepted them at once, because of the similarity in climate of the two areas of Asia.

In the beginning, Kampō was available only to the aristocracy, because of the prices and the small number of doctors who could practice Kampō. It was not until the fifteenth century, when the middle class began to make itself prominent, that Kampō became a popular medical treatment among the common people. For the next 300 years it made remarkable progress. It was altered many times over from its original Chinese methods and was adapted to the Japanese physical and mental environment.

During the eighteenth century, Rampō, or Western medicine, began to rival Kampō in popularity, and Kampō started its downward trend. In 1858, a smallpox plague broke out in Japan, and a vaccine was brought from Holland to curb smallpox. It was miraculously effective in controlling that plague, while Kampō was unable to cure the victims of smallpox, so Western medicine became dominant in Japan.

Two additional aspects of Kampō are acupuncture and moxibustion. The basic idea of the two stimulative remedies are explained simply. If a special stimulation is effected on a proper point on the body, the body will respond by changing, and this in turn will have an effect on the locale of the malady. If the stimulant is in excess, the reaction will only have an unfavorable influence on the ailment. However, if the stimulant is just right, it will promote the body's inherent power to cure and facilitate its own recovery.

Acupuncture stimulates the body by thrusting a pointed needle into the flesh. The needle is made of gold, silver, iron, or imitation platinum. It is very thin and ranges from 0.004 – 0.012 inches in diameter. The process is not at all painful if the acupuncturist is an experienced practitioner.

The method for the thrust of the needle into the skin varies. It can be slight, deep, kept in a long time or momentarily; removed by flipping, pushing, and pulling repeatedly. It can be inserted vertically or slanted. Acupuncture has been introduced into the mid-European countries and the U.S., where it is under study.

Moxibustion is the method of giving thermal stimulation on the skin. Moxa is the white hair on the back of mugwort leaves, dried, compressed, and formed into cones or sticks. The moxa, which is easy to handle, burns instantly and evenly. It varies in size with the application, but the usual size is about the size of a grain of rice. The burning temperature for moxa is from 60 degrees Celsius to 100 degrees Celsius, and it can be increased by fanning to control the stimulation. The scientific value of moxibustion is said to improve the blood circulation and increase the white corpuscles.

The points at which to apply these local stimulation remedies have been fixed by thousands of years of experience. The vital points are known as *keiketsu* and are located on the external surface of the body, on the face, palms, and even the soles of the feet. They are divided into groups called *keiraku* and linked by tracks. The keiraku play an important role in the treatment. By locating the related points in the keiraku, a toothache can be cured through the stimulation of the points in the limbs. Stomach ache and gallstones can be dealt with by stimulating points on the back.

Although Kampō is not as effective as modern medicine, especially in social, preventive, and surgical areas, it can effect treatments impossible for modern medicines. No Kampō school of instruction is available. One has to learn under a Kampō practitioner and learn the Kampō techniques singularly. The main area where these trainees fail is the lack of objectivity in their working with patients. This is the reason why Kampō does not have a place with modern Western medicines. It cannot be transmitted by textbooks and its scriptures alone. Its fatal flaw lies in its inability to reach any objectivity.

When we speak of spiritual healing, we mean the healing of the spirit within, which is expressed out-

232

wardly and visibly as improved physical conditions. In many instances this is the curing of disease or the healing of injuries. It is not anything magical, as many people think. It is a spontaneous thing which reaches out from the healer and touches the victim, making him whole again.

We live in power tides and cycles, but few seem to know this, and until we begin to learn this, suffering will be our lot. These tides and cycles are part of the cosmogony, the relative movements of complicated systems of planetary chains and rounds, races, and subraces. In other words, we have tides of power which lift one race above the other in the history of the world, and cycles which affect this particular race's affairs while in power. This is also true of the individual, and he must learn how to live with these tides of power and their cycles. Within the races, these cycles, or rounds of the orbits, come in about the fourth through the sixth generation, but it depends on the original stock of the founders and related peoples. If the race stays together, it is possible for an empire or a nation to last for many generations. As long as each group, family, and race holds together as a tight cell in society, they are practically invincible.

These cycles of nature which strike the individual, family, groups, and races are cycles of the peak of power tides or extreme good health, happiness, and prosperity, or the opposite.

The destruction of a family's longevity can also come about through vice and dissipation, which leads to a downgrading of health and satisfactory old age. Anyone who is low in his mental and physical

233

health will naturally go lower when the psychic and physical cycles of the negative types hit him.

The greatest vices which can bring about the downfall of a family are drugs and alcohol. We have plenty of knowledge, research, and communication on the results of drug abuse, but few people pay much attention. People can play dangerous games with their health at almost any time. It comes back to the one thing which is basic in all life: we are responsible to a large degree for maintaining our health. We are aware that LSD can affect the chromosomes and genes. Most drugs tend to be damaging to the brain cells, and more than one pleasure seeker has died from the aftereffects of a session with drugs.

Man does not understand that so much of his physical health will originate in other planes — the Astral, Causal, Mental, or Soul regions. All he can think about is that some biochemist's medicine will cure his ailments or that a psychologist is going to free his mental realm of its aberrations.

What we are mainly concerned with here is the health guidance given by the ECK Masters, the most reliable source for wisdom in any aspect of life. So often the information from the Astral Plane tells us that fasting, ascetic practices, and certain foods are best for health or spiritual growth. The ECK Masters have never gone in for any unreasonable austerities or fads in spiritual unfolding. They have always been quite reluctant to advise the average person in any of these areas because of the matter of health.

Drugs and alcohol are certainly on the list of those things which are not needed by any ECK chela, nor anyone else. This is not so much the question of karma as it is of keeping the mind clear and the body in good health. It is considered a part of one's spiritual responsibility to keep his body in good condition, so that he can do his best work, using the body as an instrument. For this reason the Living ECK Master always says that none are to abuse the body in any way, but to keep it in perfect health and in good tone. The physical body is man's important instrument in working out his salvation and his liberation from the Wheel of the Eighty-Four.

The popular illusion today is that the drug addict and the saint are reaching for the same experience. The addict is looking for thrills, whereas the saint is seeking the wondrous glories of God. What the addict finds is generally the lower Astral Plane, which does not seem to harbor much of anything other than wonders of the lower entities and some colors. Many of those who have been seeking a true experience of God have gone through such things and believed they had received the true glories. Many a mystic and many a saint, if one divides the categories, have had experiences in the psychic worlds, the Astral, Causal, and Mental, then had the same problems, thereafter. Each believed that he found the true heavenly kingdom.

This is the reason I have always discouraged drugs. It is a false area which the addict is led to, and he is certainly not under his own control. Furthermore, it is also detrimental to his health. When one sacrifices health in his youth, it is certain that he will not have it thereafter during his life spent on earth.

Our biggest problem is that we seldom know what is wrong with ourselves. That is, the physicians and health experts are so busy, and it is almost impossible to sit down and talk out our health problems with them. And in many cases it might be best not to discuss such matters. This is the same problem that the Living ECK Master has with so many people who are trying to bypass physical plane living and enter into the heavenly worlds in hopes of healing, good health, and a full purse. If he said what was really on his mind then it might defeat the individual completely. That person might go into a deep depression and not be able to pull out of it. In other words, it is best not to say anything at particular times because of such reactions.

This is not a question of being dishonest with the consultee but it is a matter of perhaps giving him a little longer to live by not putting a certain amount of worry into his mind.

Then again, if telling the afflicted that something is wrong arouses him into some action to take care of himself, the information can be given out, all or in parts, to suit the purpose. It depends on the person and his nature as to whether he should have full knowledge of what his ailments might be.

It is said that one of the best foods we can eat is an egg, which contains both cholesterol and its synergist; it also contains lecithin in abundance. The egg is a good food as it contains all the factors necessary to nourish life. It is easily obtained and easy for anyone to cook. It is best to have hard-boiled, soft-boiled, or poached eggs. Fried eggs are hard to digest if they are cooked in bacon grease or butter. A raw egg contains avidin which combines with and inactivates biotin (one of the essential B vitamins) in the intestinal tract, but when an egg is cooked at a temperature of over 160 degrees Fahrenheit, the avidin is destroyed. On the other hand, if the egg is heated over 212 degrees Fahrenheit, the heat will damage the sulfur-bearing amino acids, and the egg becomes less useful to the body.

Eggs are probably the most nutritious staple food available to man. Milk is claimed to be the second most nutritious food, according to certain health authorities. Liver, lean meats, and cottage cheese are rated high among nutritious foods.

If one is thinking of dieting to lose weight, he will find that problems arise. For example, take the all-protein diet in which one has an intake of lean meats and supposedly few fats and carbohydrates. The whole problem here, if one is not careful, is the drinking of water to flush out the daily waste matter of the body. Some of these diets call for eight ten-ounce glasses of water daily. This diet will take off weight, but one must be careful not to let the vitamin and mineral balance of his body be disturbed on such a regimen. He should consume multivitamin tablets daily along with a mineral complex, in order to keep up this balance within his body. Otherwise, the diet does him little good, because he is losing these all-important essentials, and his health will decrease. This is why anyone who wishes to diet should be careful to watch those things which might be injurious to his health.

Old age can be reversed in many people. A strong regimen of vitamin injections, good nutrition, vitamin supplements, and minerals can alter the processes of old age. When the aging of the glands, especially the pituitary, is halted or reversed, one begins to feel the turn toward youth again. The feeling of persecution which often comes with old age is given up, and the individual starts thinking of things to do. Gray hair and wrinkles start to disappear, and in their place come glossy hair, smooth and wrinkleless skin, the signs of youth.

But to have youth, one must also have willpower and imagination, using both to secure a place in a world which assesses the energies of younger people more fit for performance.

12

Health as an Aid in
Spiritual Growth

Those who are vitally interested in health should try to keep to an all-purpose diet consisting of essential nerve-building vitamins, blood-building minerals, gland-stimulating protein, and the hormone-nourishing unsaturated fatty acids, as well as all the other necessary ingredients which give good health to the body.

Illness or disease is created by multiple causes. We seldom think about the individual activities of the cells and groups of cells, but we do know that the body cells are kept in good health by the ingress of inorganic cell salts.

The mineral salts are very important to the functions of the cells of the human body. According to the biochemic system of medicine, there are several basic tissue cell salts which are necessary to the human body, either to ward off illnesses or to maintain general good health.

These tissue cell salts are as follows: (1) Calcarea

239

Fluorica (Fluoride of Lime); (2) Calcarea Phosphorica (Phosphate of Lime); (3) Calcarea Sulphurica (Sulphate of Lime); (4) Ferrum Phosphoricum (Phosphate of Iron); (5) Kali Muriaticum (Chloride of Potash); (6) Kali Phosphoricum (Phosphate of Potash); (7) Kali Sulphuricum (Sulphate of Potash); (8) Magnesia Phosphorica (Phosphate of Magnesia); (9) Natrum Muriaticum (Chloride of Soda); (10) Natrum Phosphoricum (Phosphate of Soda); (11) Natrum Sulphuricum (Sulphate of Soda); and (12) Silicea (Silica). These were isolated by intense research by Dr. W.H. Schuessler over 100 years ago, and his analysis seems to have been successful.

The function activated by each of these salts balances the physiological needs of the body and its vital organs and tissues. If the body does not have the proper intake of various mineral salts in the daily diet, the mineral imbalance will cause certain disorders.

The mineral salts named above act upon the physical system in various ways:

Calcarea Fluorica is found in the surface of the bones, in the enamel of the teeth, and in the elastic fibers of the skin, muscular tissue, and blood vessels. Calcarea Fluorica is said to be the remedy for diseases affecting the surface of the bones and the enamel of the teeth. A deficiency of Calcarea Fluorica results in a loosened condition of the elastic fibers, including dilation of the blood vessels, hemorrhoids, varicose veins, hardened glands, and cracks in the skin.

Calcarea Phosphorica is a constitutent of the bones, teeth, connective tissue, blood corpuscles,

240

and the gastric juices. It unites with the organic substance albumin, giving solidity to the bones, building the teeth, and entering into the secretions of the body, like the blood and gastric juices. Bone structure is fifty-seven percent Calcarea Phosphorica, and without it no bone can be formed.

Calcarea Phosphorica uses albumin as a cement to build bone structure. It enters into the formation of teeth which makes it a good supplement in childhood to build good teeth. It also plays an important part in assimilation and digestion. It is closely allied with Magnesia Phosphorica and is frequently given in alternation with it as a remedy in some ailments.

Calcarea Phosphorica is used to treat bone diseases, whether inherited or due to nutritional deficiency. It aids the union of fractured bones and is a remedy in anemia and chlorosis, and, in the young, aids the growth of teeth. It is also useful in building up new blood corpuscles after an acute disease.

Calcarea Sulphurica is found in the epithelial skin cells and in the blood. It is a preventive of cell disintegration and suppuration. A deficiency of Calcarea Sulphurica allows suppuration to continue, and wounds are slow to heal. It works well with Silicea in healing of catarrhs, boils, ulcers, etc.

Ferrum Phosphoricum is a remedy for inflammatory and feverish conditions. It is found in the blood where it gives the corpuscles their reddish color. It gives strength to the walls of the arteries and blood vessels. Ferrum Phosphoricum is said to be the most essential cell salt of all, for it is thought to be the healing agency for body inflammation. It is also used in cases of abnormal conditions of the blood corpuscles and in cases of trouble with muscular tissue.

Kali Muriaticum unites with albumin and forms fibrin, which is found in every tissue of the body with exception of the bones. A deficiency of this cell salt will cause a discharge of a white, thick, sticky substance from the mucous membranes and a heavy white or gray coating of the tongue.

Kali Muriaticum is also a remedy for catarrhal conditions, and it is used in controlling spasmodic croup, diarrhea, and bronchitis. In conditions associated with deficiency of Kali Muriaticum, the blood tends to thicken and form clots. Kali Muriaticum is often referred to as the liver salt, because of its action on this vital organ of the body. It helps maintain the fluidity of the blood and it stimulates the flow of the bile.

Kali Phosphoricum is a component of all the tissues and fluids of the body, mostly of the brain and nerve cells. It is known to be one of the best nutrients of the nervous system, and it has an antiseptic action which hinders decay of the tissues.

A deficiency of Kali Phosphoricum produces brain fatigue, mental depression, irritability, fearfulness, timidity, lack of nervous energy. It is good in overcoming muscular debility, following acute diseases which are associated with distribution of nervous energies to the vital organs. One of the most prominent symptoms of a deficiency of Kali Phosphoricum is prostration, along with sluggish conditions of the mind and an exhausted mental state following exertion or emotional strain.

Kali Sulphuricum is a carrier of oxygen to the cells of the skin. The oxygen in the lungs is taken up by the iron in the blood and carried to every cell in the body by the respective actions of Kali Sulphuricum and Ferrum Phosphoricum.

A deficiency of Kali Sulphuricum will cause a lack of oxygen in the skin and in the epithelial cells and will give rise to symptoms of chilliness, shifting inflammatory pain, and a desire for cool air. Kali Sulphuricum is a remedy for skin troubles. It promotes perspiration, handles dandruff problems, catarrh of the stomach and bowels, and diarrhea.

Magnesia Phosphorica is an antispasmodic and works chiefly with the delicate white fibers of the nerves and muscles. It uses albumin and water to form the transparent fluid which nourishes these fibers.

A deficiency of Magnesia Phosphorica in the fiber allows it to contract, to produce spasms and cramps. When this contraction takes place there is pressure on the sensory nerves which gives rise to sharp, shooting, darting, neuralgic pains in any part of the body.

Natrum Muriaticum is the constituent of every liquid and solid part of the body. It regulates the degree of moisture in the cells by virtue of its property of attracting and distributing water. The body is composed of about seventy percent water, which in the absence of Natrum Muriaticum would be inert and useless. Any deficiency of the cell salt causes an imbalance of water in the human organism. The patient will have a watery, bloated appearance, will be languid, drowsy, and inclined to have a dulled mental outlook on life.

Natrum Muriaticum regulates the quantity of water entering into the composition of the blood corpuscles. Natrum Muriaticum also controls the production of hydrochloric acid, regulates the density of the fluids which surround the tissue cells, and promotes the activity of changes in the tissues.

Natrum Phosphoricum is necessary to the blood, muscles, nerves, and the intercellular fluids. It also splits up the lactic acid into carbonic acid and water, and it is the specialized remedy where there is an excess of acid in the system. Any acid condition in the body system gives rise to rheumatism, digestive upsets, intestinal disorders, and has an adverse effect upon the assimilation of food in the body. Natrum Phosphoricum helps regulate the consistency of bile and is good in treating colic, sick headaches, and gastric disturbances.

One of the functions of Natrum Phosphoricum is that of assisting in the absorption of water, which is quite different from that of Natrum Muriaticum, which distributes water, and Natrum Sulphuricum, which eliminates surplus water from the body. The presence of these three tissue salts in the body controls the manner in which the body fluids behave.

Natrum Phosphoricum serves to emulsify the fatty acids which irritate the digestive system after eating fatty or greasy foods. It corrects gastric troubles in small children who suffer from an excess of lactic acid from milk and sugar.

Natrum Sulphuricum is found only in the intercellular fluids. Its principal function is to regulate the quantity of water in the tissues, blood, and fluids of the body. It has an attachment for water, and it eliminates any excess from the bile.

Natrum Sulphuricum splits the lactic acid into carbonic acid and water, leaving a residue of water to be removed from the body system. At the same time, Natrum Sulphuricum starts removing the excess water from the body.

A lack of Natrum Sulphuricum will create excess bile flow, jaundice, biliousness, and diarrhea. Such symptoms are irritated by the use of water in any form, that is, by living in low, marshy places, damp buildings, basements, or by eating water plants, fish, and similar foods.

Silicea is found abundantly in the vegetable kingdom, especially in grasses, grains, and palms. It is present in the blood, bile, skin, hair, and nails. It is also a constituent of the connective tissue, bones, nerve sheaths, and mucous membranes. A lack of it shows up when there is a deficient assimilation of food in the body.

One of the secrets of recharging the body lies in a raw fruit and vegetable diet. The Japanese people, who seem to have a longevity greater than ours as a race, eat a great deal of raw fish. A diet of this nature with raw fruit and vegetables can revitalize the entire system of the human body.

There are many Japanese who believe in a vegetarian diet. Since the sixth century when it was first introduced into Japan, the Buddhist religion, which came to have a strong hold on the Japanese, forbade the killing and eating of animal flesh. Despite this, people consumed much fish and bird meat, along with a few vegetables. Later, with the spread of Zen during the twelfth century, the eating of vegetables, both raw and cooked, supplemented with fish, became prominent in the Japanese diet.

This is quite like the ECK diet, which has been used in the Katsupari Monastery in northern Tibet. Because the emphasis is put upon raw foods, cooked vegetables, fish and poultry, fruits and seeds, many of the diseases which afflict modern man, such as stomach ulcer, arteriosclerosis, and cancer, are unheard of among those who are in the monastery. They acquire vegetables, herbs, vitamins, and minerals from their true sources.

Raw fish, especially the way the Japanese prepare it as sashimi, is a good, nutritious protein. It is also easy for people of almost any age to digest.

The best types of fish served raw in Japan are: First, the river fish — carp, crucian carp, trout; second, the best in the sea — bonito, flounder, mullet, mackerel, pompano, sea bream, snipefish, squid, tuna, and yellowtail; and third, the shellfish — the ark shell, clam, cockle, abalone, oyster, and crab.

It is never advisable to eat raw fish except at a good restaurant where it has been properly prepared. Parasites can be eliminated by a skillful cook. No public restaurant in Japan is allowed to operate without health department licenses, so generally one can be safe in eating raw fish there; but to try to prepare raw fish in one's own home is not at all good, for there are always the dangers of allergies and parasites.

An excellent meal which the Japanese serve as a light, simple snack or luncheon is called *ochazuke,* a tasty dish of rice steeped in tea with seaweed on top. Seaweed is a good food somewhat neglected in the Western world, but we are gradually learning that the sea furnishes many more herbs, vitamins, and minerals than we formerly believed.

246

The reason most people are tired is that they lack enzymes in their bodies. The food which they eat cannot be digested and utilized, and instead, becomes waste matter and turns to toxins and poisons.

Enzymes offer the key to longevity, as discussed in chapter 2. Sprouted seeds are among our richest sources of enzymes. Another excellent source is the red potato, which contains vitamin C and a very powerful enzyme, tyrosinase. In England, they have set up youth rejuvenation clinics where the fresh juice of raw red potatoes is used every few hours, and within two weeks the person is said to look ten to twenty years younger. Do not use potato sprouts or potatoes that have a green coloration under the peeling. The sprouts and green portions contain an enzyme that will lock up the digestive system so it cannot process (digest) proteins and will make one very sick.

These invisible workers, the enzymes, seem to be able to neutralize the basic causes of aging in the body and help retain its youthful qualities. The best way of putting additional enzymes into the body is to eat fruit, properly grown vegetables, certain meats, and grains and seeds.

It has been found that vinegar and spice-laden dressings used on salads, generally destroy or render the enzymes useless. Enzymes are also destroyed in the processing and canning of various vegetables and meats.

Wheat kernels contain the important enzymes of amylase and protease. Grinding the wheat into flour does not harm the enzymes, but the heat used in baking the flour into bread does destroy them. Butter has no enzymes, because the heat used to pasteurize the

247

cream from which the butter is made destroys them. Canned juices may be rich in vitamins, but the enzymes were destroyed when the juices were heated and poured into the cans. Generally, breakfast foods have few enzymes which have survived the roasting, baking, and packing.

All sugars, including the variety known as raw sugar, do not have many enzymes, because sugar is subjected to a prolonged boiling. The original cane sugar was rich in enzymes, but these disappeared when sugar was boiled for human consumption.

We treat our animals better than ourselves, because they get raw products to eat, including cane stalks, while we get processed products. Boiling potatoes, meat, and leafy vegetables in water will bring about a complete destruction of enzymes.

It is important that one understand that longevity is based upon the enzymes. Much study is being done on the subject by medical researchers the world over.

Good diet is a proper cure for depression cycles, said to be the world's most widespread emotional illness. Depression cycles are said to hit millions of people yearly in the United States alone. The most common symptoms are sadness, constant fatigue, loss of interest in social life, self-neglect, and insomnia. People who are affected with depression cycles in an extreme way and who find themselves in what can be said to be an emotional binge, should take a good look at their diet.

It has been reported that these depressions may be the manifestation of deficiencies of B vitamins, especially B_{12}. The average person can help to offset B vitamin deficiency by eating brewer's yeast and liver.

Another culprit responsible for depressive states and similar illnesses is the low blood sugar problem. The most important nutrient required by the brain is glucose, a sugar, and when it is not available, depression appears. It is a paradox, but too much sugar in the diet makes for a low blood sugar problem in the body. When too many sweets are eaten, the blood becomes loaded with sugar and may cause diabetes.

In place of excessive sweets and starches, one can change his diet to include fresh broccoli, brussels sprouts, cabbage, cauliflower, carrots, and similar vegetables. He can also eat unsweetened fruits, such as apples, apricots, berries, grapefruits, and bananas. Sugar-rich soft drinks should be cut off the list, along with coffee, because caffeine affects the sugar metabolism of the body.

Another problem of a similar nature can be a depressed state in which the patient hears voices, becomes tense, nervous, and fatigued. Sometimes doctors put the person with such problems on niacin, or vitamin B_3, and the difficulty clears up in a relatively short period of time. Others have stated that vitamins C, B_1, B_6, B_{12}, and folic acid will take care of this problem.

Oftentimes when people are burdened with the negative emotions, niacin and other vitamin B nutrients will resolve the dour attitude. It is known among health authorities that illnesses of this nature can result when either environmental factors or chemicals produced in the body upset the ratio of various molecules carried by the blood to the brain. Any deficiency of nutrients needed to nourish the brain can also cause an imbalance in the body and mind.

249

It is the opinion of some that the proper functioning of the brain requires the right chemicals in the right amounts. The kind of chemical molecules which control the brain's activities, along with the nervous system's health, have an incredibly significant influence upon the functions of these organs. Most people are aware that a mere speck of LSD entering the bloodstream through the stomach will radically upset the functions of the brain for at least twelve hours.

This is why I have spoken against fasting and other particular ideas which concern the nutrition of the body. If one is deficient in several nutrients which are necessary for the body health, it is possible that he can fall into psychoneurosis and similar types of emotional disturbances. For example, it is claimed that a lack of thiamine can bring ideas of persecution, mental confusion, and bad memory. A deficiency of riboflavin can cause depression, visual disturbances, disordered thinking, and inability to concentrate. A lack of niacin may result in unreasonable fears, anxiety, mania, hallucinations, and dementia. Insufficient pyridoxine may bring on convulsions and irritability.

All important food factors — proteins, nucleic acids, vitamins, minerals, and enzymes — work together to help keep man more youthful, regardless of his age.

According to important studies, the vitamin which one can most depend upon to help him avoid the hallmarks of old age — loss of teeth, shrinking in stature, wrinkling of skin, and other symptoms of that dreaded thing we know as old age — is said to be vitamin C.

While vitamin E is considered one of the best for keeping the body in good shape, it is now believed that vitamin C is likely to be of great help in aiding the body to renew itself. This vitamin gives strength to the body to resist and to recover from the destructive attacks of disease.

More vitamin C is needed as one gets older. It is a requisite for the formation of collagen, an essential protein in bone, cartilage, connective tissue, and skin. The need for regenerating collagen is the prime reason that vitamin C requirements increase with age.

Some people need more vitamins, minerals, and enzymes than others. The mistake which nutritionists make as a fundamental error is attempting to set up a uniform standard for all people. It is not possible to put everybody on a standard diet, and this may be the cause of breakdowns in the physical systems of many people who try to follow such standards. What is one man's poison is another man's meat, so the old saying goes. Each person must study himself and see just what is best for his own body and mind on a daily intake of foods, and which will give him the best nutrients to benefit his energy and capacity for good living.

One of the things which many people do not understand is that chronic bowel problems brought on by poor choice of foods is a major cause of varicose veins, according to reports from health authorities. In Britain, at least ten percent of the population suffers from varicose veins. This means that one should look to the simplicity of diets having reasonable amounts of meats, fish, poultry, fresh eggs, whole grain bread, nuts, raisins, salads, and vegetables.

Most people's physical and diet problems started when they were children, especially at school age. Those who ate large amounts of sweets were bound to eat little else, and the lack of good food soon began to show itself in weakness and disease. When they reached middle age or old age, their difficulties became more prominent, unless there had been an attempt to remedy the situation.

One will not be able to bring about results overnight through correction of diet. Although there can be some immediate improvement, the dramatic changes will usually take longer than most people will want to wait. Only patience and proper diet will bring results.

In their children's formative years, parents have a great influence which must be channeled toward giving the children good eating habits. These habits can keep them healthy through their respective lives. Since parents are the source of their children's food supply, the parents must give them only what they should have. Apples must be shown to be better for snacks than a piece of cake. Let the child drink fruit juice instead of soda. If this can be done, at least half of the battle to get the child to eat good, nourishing food is won. At least it will give him an early chance to learn how to make selections of foods which will preserve his good health.

Many things have been left unsaid in this book. Good health is every man's right, but no man will keep it if he is careless as to what he feeds his body and mind daily.

Appendix

Herbs and Their Botanical Names

Common Name	Latin Name
A	
Adam and Eve Root	*Aplectrum hyemale*
alder	*Prinos spp.*
alder, black	*Prinos verticillatus* (Linn.)
alfalfa	*Medicago sativa* (Linn.)
alkanet	*Alkanna tinctoria* (Tausch.)
allspice	*Pimenta dioica*
almond, sweet	*Amygdalus communis var. dulcis*
almond, bitter	*Amygdalus communis var. amara*
alumroot	*Heuchera americana*
American centaury	*Sabatia angularis*
anemone	*Anemone spp.*
angelica	*Angelica archangelica* (Linn.)
anise	*Pimpinella anisum* (Linn.)
annatto	*Bixa orellana* (Linn.)
apple	*Malus spp.*
apple mint	*Mentha rotundifolia* and *M. gentilis*

apricot	*Prunus armeniaca* (Linn.)
arbutus, trailing	*Epigaea repens* (Linn.)
artichoke	*Cynara scolymus*
asparagus	*Asparagus officinalis*

B

balm	*Melissa officinalis* (Linn.)
balm of Gilead fir	*Abies balsamea* (Linn.)
balsam of Gilead	*Commiphora opobalsamum*
barley	*Hordeum vulgare*
basil, sweet	*Ocimum basilicum* (Linn.)
bearberry	*Arctostaphylos uva-ursi*
beets	*Beta spp.*
bell pepper	*Capsicum frutescens grossum*
benzoin	*Styrax benzoin* (Dry.)
bergamot mint	*Monarda didyma*
betel nut	*Areca catechu* (Linn.)
bethroot	*Trillium pendulum* (Willd.)
bilberry	*Vaccinium myrtillus* (Linn.)
birch, bark	*Betula alba*
blackberry	*Rubus fructicosus*
black root	*Leptandra virginica* (Nutt.)
black willow	*Salyx nigra* (March)
bloodroot	*Sanguinaria candesis* (Linn.)
blueberry	*Vaccinium ssp.*
boneset	*Eupatorium perfoliatum* (Linn.)
broccoli	*Brassica oleracea italica*
broom tops	*Cystisus scoparius* (Linn.)
Brussels sprouts	*Brassica oleracea gemmifera*
buckeye	*Aesculus spp.*
buckthorn, alder	*Rhamnus frangula* (Linn.)
buckthorn, common	*Rhamnus cathartica*
buckwheat	*Polygonum fagopyrum*
bugle, common	*Ajuga reptans* (Linn.)
burdock	*Arctium lappa* (Linn.)
butterbur	*Petasites vulgaris* (Desf.)

254

butterfly weed	*Asclepias tuberose* (Linn.)
butternut	*Juglans cinerea* (Linn.)

C

cabbage	*Brassica oleracea capitata*
calamint	*Calamintha officinalis* (Moench)
calamus	*Acorus calamus* (Linn.)
calumba root	*Jateorhiza calumba* (Miers)
Canada snakeroot	see ginger, wild
cape mint	*Mentha capensis*
caraway	*Carum carvi* (Linn.)
cardamom seed	*Elettaria cardamomum* (Maton)
carob	*Ceratonia siliqua* (Linn.)
carrot	*Daucus carota*
carrot, wild	*Daucus carota* (Linn.)
cascara sagrada	*Rhamnus purshiana*
cassia	*Cinnamomum cassia* (Blume)
catnip	*Nepeta cataria* (Linn.)
cauliflower	*Brassica oleracea botrytis*
cayenne pepper	*Capsicum frutescens longum*
celery	*Apium graveolens* (Linn.)
chamomile	
English/Roman	*Anthemis nobilis* (Linn.)
German/Hungarian	*Matricaria chamomilla* (Linn.)
chard	*Beta vulgaris cicla*
cherry	*Prunus spp.*
cherry, wild, bark	*Prunus serotina* (Ehrh.)
chia	*Salvia columbariae* (Linn.)
chicory root	*Cichorium intybus* (Linn.)
chickweed	*Stellaria media* (Cyrill.)
chives	*Allium schoenoprasum*
chocolate root	*Geum rivale* (Linn.)
cinnamon	*Cinnamomum zeylanicum* (Nees.)
clary sage	*Salvia sclarea* (Linn.)
clover, red	*Trifolium pratense* (Linn.)
clover, sweet	*Meliotus officinalis* (Linn.)

255

cloves	*Eigemoa caryophyllata* (Thumb.)
cleavers	*Galium aparine*
coconut	*Cocos nucifera*
coffee	*Coffea spp.*
cohosh, blue	*Caulophyllum thalictroides* (Mich.)
coltsfoot	*Tussilago farfara*
comfrey	*Symphytum officinale*
coriander	*Coriandrum sativum* (Linn.)
corn	*Zea mays* (Linn.)
couch grass	*Agropyrum repens* (Beauv.)
cucumber, skin	*Cucumis sativa* (Linn.)
cumin seed	*Cuminum cyminum* (Linn.)
curled mint	*Mentha crispa*
cyclamen	*Cyclamen hederaefolium*

D

damiana	*Turnera aphrodisiaca* (Willd.)
dandelion	*Taraxacum officinale* (Weber)
date	*Phoenix dactylifera*
deer's tongue	*Liatris odoratissima* (Willd.)
desert herb	*Ephedra spp.*
devil's bit scabious	*Scabiosa succisa*
devil's shoestrings	*Tephrosia virginiana*
docks,	
yellow or curled	*Rumex crispus*
dog rose	*Rosa canina*
dulse	*Rhodymenia palmata* (Linn.)

E

eggplant	*Solanum melongena*
eglantine	*Rosa rubiginosa*
elder	*Sambucus nigra* (Linn.)
elder,	
dwarf American	*Aralia hispida*
elecampane root	*Inula helenium* (Linn.)

256

endive	*Chicorium endiva*
eryngo (sea holly)	*Eryngium maritinum*
eyebright	*Euphrasia officinalis* (Linn.)

F

fennel seed	*Foeniculum vulgare* (Gaert.)
fenugreek	*Trigonella foenum-graecum* (Linn.)
figs	*Ficus carica* (Linn.)
five-finger grass	*Potentilla reptans* (Linn.)
flax, seed	*Linum usitatissimum* (Linn.)
flax, mountain, seed	*Linum catharitcum* (Linn.)
fo-ti-tieng	*Hydrocotyle asiatica minor*
frankincense	*Boswellia thurfura*

G

garlic	*Allium sativum* (Linn.)
gentian	*Gentiana lutea* (Linn.)
ginger, Jamaica	*Zingiber officinale* (Rosc.)
wild ginger	*Asarum canadense* (Linn.)
ginseng, American	*Panax quinquefolius* (Linn.)
ginseng, Asiatic	*Panax schinseng*
golden maidenhair	*Polytrichum vulgare*
goldenrod	*Solidago virgaurea* (Linn.)
goldenseal	*Hydrastis canadensis* (Linn.)
gotu kola	*Hydrocotyle asiatica*
grains of paradise	*Aframomum melegueta*
granadilla	*Passiflora incarnata* (Linn.)
grapefruit	*Citrus paradisi*
gravel plant	*Epigaea repens* (Linn.)
ground ivy	*Nepeta hederacea*
grumichama	*Eugenia dombeyi* or *E. brasiliensis*
guarana	*Paullinia cupana* (H.B. & K.)

H

hawthorn	*Crataegus oxyacantha* (Linn.)
hemlock	*Tsuga canadensis* (Linn.)

hemp	*Cannabis sativa*
henna	*Lawsonia alba* (Lank.)
hops	*Humulus lupulus* (Linn.)
horehound	*Marrubium vulgare* (Linn.)
horsemint	*Mentha sylvestris* (Linn.)
horsemint, American	*Monarda punctata* (Linn.)
horseradish root	*Cochlearia armoracia* (Linn.)
horsetails	*Equisetum arvense*
	E. hyemale
	E. maximum
	E. sylvaticum
hyssop	*Hyssopus officinalis* (Linn.)

I

Iceland moss	*Cetraria islandica* (Ach.)
Irish moss	*Chondrus Crispus* (Stackh.)

J

jagua	*Maximiliana regia*
jasmine	*Jasminum officinale* (Linn.)
juniper	*Juniperus communis* (Linn.)

K

kale	*Brassica oleracea acephala*
kamala	*Mallotus philippinensis* (Muell.)
kava kava	*Piper methysticum* (Forst.)
kelp	*Phaephyta*
knotgrass	*Polyganum aviculare* (Linn.)
kola nut	*Cola spp.*

L

lady's slipper	*Cypripedium pubescens* (Willd.)
lavender	*Lavandula vera*
leek	*Allium porrum*
lemon	*Citrus limonum* (Risso.)
lemon balm	*Melissa officinalis* (Linn.)
lentils	*Lens culinaris*

leptotaenia	*Lomatium dissectum multifidum*
lettuce	*Lactuca spp.*
lettuce,	
head, iceberg	*Lactuca sativa var.capitata*
lettuce, wild	*Lactuca virosa* (Linn.)
licorice	*Glycyrrhiza glabra* (Linn.)
life root	*Senecio aureus* (Linn.)
lily, white pond	*Nymphaea odorata* (Soland)
lovage	*Levisticum officinale* (Koch.)

M

madder	*Rubia tinctorum* (Linn.)
maidenhair fern	*Adiantum capillus-veneris* (Linn.)
malva, blue	*Malva sylvestris* (Linn.)
mandrake	*Atropa mandragora*
mango	*Mangifera indica*
marigold	*Calendula officinalis* (Linn.)
marjoram, pot	*Origanum onites*
marjoram, sweet	*Origanum marjoram* (Linn.)
may apple root	*Podophyllum peltatum* (Linn.)
meadowsweet	*Spiraea ulmaria*
mistletoe	*Viscum album* (Linn.)
motherwort	*Leonurus cardiaca* (Linn.)
mountain ash	*Pyrus domestica*
mullein	*Verbascum spp.*
mugwort	*Artemisia vulgaris* (Linn.)
mung bean	*Phaseolus aureus*
musk root	*Ferula sumbul* (Hooker Fil.)
mustard, green	*Brassica japonica, B. juncea*
mustard, black	*Brassica nigra* (Linn.)
mustard, white	*Brassica hirta*
myrrh	*Commiphora myrrha* (Holmes)
myrtle	*Myrtaceae*

N

nettles	*N.O. Urticaceae*
nettles, greater	*Urtica dioica* (Linn.)

O

oak, English	*Quercus robur* (Linn.)
oak, white, bark	*Quercus alba*
oat	*Avena sativa*
olives	*Olea europaea*
onion	*Allium cepa* (Linn.)
orange	*Citrus aurantium* (Linn.)
Oregon grape	*Mahonia aquifolium*
orrisroot	*Iris florentina*

P

papaya	*Carica papaya*
paprika	*Capsicum annuum* (Linn.)
parsley	*Petroselinum crispum*
parsnip	*Pastinaca sativa*
passion flower	*Passiflora incarnata* (Linn.)
peach	*Prunus persica* (Stokes)
peanut	*Arachis hypogaea* (Linn.)
pearl-flowered life everlasting	*Antennaria margaritiaceum*
pecan	*Carya illinoensis*
pennyroyal	*Mentha pulegium* (Linn.)
peppermint	*Mentha piperita* (Sm.)
pimiento	*Capsicum frutescens*
pimpernel	*Anagallis arvensis* (Linn.)
pine, white	*Pinus strobus* (Linn.)
pinguin	*Bromelia pinguin*
pipsissewa	*Chimaphila umbellata* (Linn.)
pitanga	*Eugenia uniflora*
plantain	*Plantago major*
pomegranate	*Punica granatum* (Linn.)
poppy seed	*Papaver somniferum* (Linn.)
potato, red	*Solanum tuberosum*
primrose	*Primula vulgaris* (Huds.)
privet	*Ligustrum vulgare*
psyllium seed	*Plantago psyllium* (Linn.)

pumpkin	*Cucurbita pepo*
purslane	*Portulaca oleracea*

Q

quassia chips	*Picraena excelsa* (Lindl.)
queen's delight	*Stillingia sylvatica* (Linn.)

R

radish	*Raphanus sativus*
raisin	*Vitas vinifera*
raspberry	*Rubus idaeus*
rest harrow	*Ononis arvensis*
rhubarb	*Rheum rhaponticum*
rice, brown	*Oryza sativa*
rose	*Rosa spp.*
rosemary	*Rosmarinus officinalis* (Linn.)
rue	*Ruta graveolens* (Linn.)
rye	*Secale cereale*

S

saffron	*Crocus sativus*
sage	*Salvia officinalis* (Linn.)
saguaro cactus	*Carnegiea gigantea*
St. John's bread	*Ceratonia siliqua* (Linn.)
Saint-John's-wort	*Hypericum perforatum* (Linn.)
salep	*Orchis spp.*
sandalwood	*Santalum album* (Linn.)
sanicle	*Sanicula europaea* (Linn.)
sarsaparilla	*Smilax officinalis*
satyrion	*Orchis maculata* (Linn.)
saunders, red	*Pterocarpus santalinus*
saw palmetto	*Sarenoa serrulata* (Hook, F.)
scouring rush	*Equisetum hyemale* (Linn.)
seneca root	*Polygala senega* (Linn.)
senna pod	*Cassia acutifolia* (Dell.)
senna, American	*Cassia marilandica*
sesame	*Sesamum indicum* (Linn.)

seven barks	*Hydrangea arborescens* (Linn.)
shave grass	*Equisetum arvense*
shepherd's purse	*Capsella bursa-pastoris*
silverweed	*Potentilla anserina*
skullcap	*Scutellaria spp.*
skunk cabbage	*Sumplocarpus foetidus*
snakehead	*Chelone glabra* (Linn.)
Solomon's seal	*Polygonatum multiflorum* (Allem.)
sorrel	*Rumex spp.*
soybean	*Glycine max*
spearmint	*Mentha spicata* (Linn.)
spikenard	*Nardostachys jatamansi*
spinach	*Spinacia oleracea* (Linn.)
squash	*Cucurbita spp.*
squaw vine	*Mitchella repens* (Linn.)
strawberries	*Fragaria vesca* (Linn.)
sumac	*Rhus glabra* (Linn.)
sunflower, seed	*Helianthus annuus*
sweet fern	*Comptonia asplenifolia*

T

taheebo	*Tecoma impetiginosa*
tamarisk	*Tamarisk gallica, var. manniferra*
tansy	*Tanacetum vulgare* (Linn.)
tea	*Camellia sinensis*
thyme, basil	*Calamintha acinos*
thyme	*Thymus vulgaris* (Linn.)
toadflax	*Linaria vulgaris*
tobacco	*Nicotiana tabacum* (Linn.)
tomato	*Lycopersicon esculentum*
tonka bean	*Dipteryx odorata* (Willd.)
tulip tree	*Liriodendron tulipifera*
turnips	*Brassica rapa*

V

valerian	*Valeriana officinalis* (Linn.)
vervain	*Verbena officinalis* (Linn.)

W

wahoo bark	*Euonymus atropurpureus*
walnut	*Juglans nigra* (Linn.)
watercress	*Nasturtium officinale*
watermelon	*Citrullus vulgaris*
water mint	*Mentha aquatica* (Linn.)
water parsnip	*Sium latifolium*
wintergreen	*Gaultheria procumbens* (Linn.)
woodruff, sweet	*Asperula odorata* (Linn.)
wormseed	*Chenopodium anthelminticum* (Bert.)
wormwood	*Artemisia absinthium* (Linn.)

Y

yams	*Dioscorea spp.*
yarrow	*Achillea millefolium* (Linn.)

Index

265

266

267

268

270

271

273

275

276

individualism, 114, 116,
    125
religious-based, 116
Vervain, 17, 175–176
Vinegar, 81, 175, 247
Virus(es), 21, 81, 82, 83
Vitamin
    A, 80, 112, 150, 173
    B, 80, 150, 155–156,
        173, 174, 202,
        248–249
    deficiency of, 115
    B₁, 205
    C, 76, 80, 173, 174,
        202, 225, 228, 247,
        249, 250, 251
    E, 202, 225, 228, 251
    X, 208

Wahoo bark, 9, 16
Walnuts, 50, 185
    hulls, 12
    leaves, 15, 38, 39
Water, 198, 225, 244
Watercress, 35, 38, 40,
    185
Watermelon, seed, 15
Weight loss, 237–238
Wheat, 18, 228
    kernels, 247
Wheat germ, 68
    oil, 50, 202, 205
Wheel of the Eighty-Four,
    122, 123, 212, 235
Wheel of Life, 181–182
Wheel of the ECK-Vidya.
    See ECK-Vidya
Wheezing, 176
Wild cherry, 14, 16

Wild lettuce, 17
Wild strawberry, 17
Wintergreen, 16
White oak, bark, 12
    root, 15
White pine, bark, 16
White pond lily, root, 15
Wormseed, 12
Wormwood, 58
Wounds, 57, 58, 178

Yarrow, 38
Yaubl Sacabi, 138, 139,
    211, 217
Yogurt, 50

Zinc, 42, 187
Zodiac signs, 123, 124

How to Study ECK Further

People want to know the secrets of life and death. In response to this need Sri Harold Klemp, today's spiritual leader of Eckankar, and Paul Twitchell, its modern-day founder, have written special monthly discourses which reveal the Spiritual Exercises of ECK—to lead Soul in a direct way to God.

Those who wish to study Eckankar can receive these special monthly discourses which give clear, simple instructions for the spiritual exercises. The first annual series of discourses is *The ECK Dream Discourses*. Mailed each month, the discourses will offer insight into your dreams and what they mean to you.

The techniques in these discourses, when practiced twenty minutes a day, are likely to prove survival beyond death. Many have used them as a direct route to Self-Realization, where one learns his mission in life. The next stage, God Consciousness, is the joyful state wherein Soul becomes the spiritual traveler, an agent for God. The underlying principle one learns is this: Soul exists because God loves It.

Membership in ECKANKAR includes:

1. Twelve monthly lessons of *The ECK Dream Discourses,* which include these titles: "Dreams—The Bridge to Heaven," "The Dream Master," "How to Interpret Your Dreams," "Dream Travel to Soul Travel," and more. You may study them alone at home or in a class with others.
2. The *Mystic World,* a quarterly newsletter with a Wisdom Note and articles by the Living ECK Master. In it are also letters and articles from students of Eckankar around the world.
3. Special mailings to keep you informed of upcoming Eckankar seminars and activities around the world, new study materials available from Eckankar, and more.
4. The opportunity to attend ECK Satsang classes and book discussions with others in your community.
5. Initiation eligibility.
6. Attendance at certain chela meetings at ECK seminars.

How to Find Out More:

Call **(612) 544-0066**, Monday through Friday, 8 a.m. to 5 p.m. central time, to find out more about how to study *The ECK Dream Discourses,* or use the coupon at the back of this book. Or write: **ECKANKAR, Att: Information, P.O. Box 27300, Minneapolis, MN 55427 U.S.A.**

Discover How You Can Receive
Spiritual Guidance and Protection

Now you can learn how to have your *own* spiritual experiences. Here are four bestsellers which can show you how to receive your own spiritual guidance, and how to use it to become the best you can be.

The Book of ECK Parables, Volume One,
Harold Klemp

Learn how to find spiritual fulfillment in everyday life from this series of over ninety light, easy-reading stories by Eckankar's spiritual leader, Sri Harold Klemp. The parables reveal secrets of Soul Travel, dreams, karma, health, reincarnation, and—most important of all—initiation into the Sound and Light of God, in everyday settings we can understand.

ECKANKAR—The Key to Secret Worlds,
Paul Twitchell

Paul Twitchell, modern-day founder of Eckankar, gives you the basics of this ancient teaching. Includes six specific Soul Travel exercises to see the Light and hear the Sound of God, plus case histories of Soul Travel. Learn to recognize yourself as Soul—and journey into the heavens of the Far Country.

The Wind of Change, Harold Klemp

What are the hidden spiritual reasons behind every event in your life? With stories drawn from his own lifelong training, Eckankar's spiritual leader shows you how to use the power of Spirit to discover those reasons. Follow him from the Wisconsin farm of his youth to a military base in Japan; from a job in Texas into the realms beyond, as he shares the secrets of Eckankar.

The Tiger's Fang, Paul Twitchell

Paul Twitchell's teacher, Rebazar Tarzs, takes him on a journey through vast worlds of Light and Sound, to sit at the feet of the spiritual Masters. Their conversations bring out the secret of how to draw closer to God—and awaken Soul to Its spiritual destiny. Many have used this book, with its vivid descriptions of heavenly worlds and citizens, to begin their own spiritual adventures.

Contact your bookstore today about these and other fine books from Illuminated Way Publishing.

Or, order direct using our toll-free number. Request a free copy of our catalog, featuring over 25 books on new age subjects.

CALL NOW
1-800-622-4408

There May Be an
ECKANKAR Study Group near You

Eckankar offers a variety of local and international activities for the spiritual seeker. With hundreds of study groups worldwide, Eckankar is near you! Many areas have Eckankar Centers where you can browse through the books in a quiet, unpressured environment, talk with others who share an interest in this ancient teaching, and attend beginning discussion classes on how to gain the attributes of Soul: wisdom, power, love, and freedom.

Around the world, Eckankar study groups offer special one-day or weekend seminars on the basic teachings of Eckankar. Check your phone book under **ECKANKAR**, or call **(612) 544-0066** for membership information and the location of the Eckankar Center or study group nearest you. Or write **ECKANKAR, Att: Information, P.O. Box 27300, Minneapolis, MN 55427 U.S.A.**

☐ Please send me information on the nearest Eckankar discussion or study group in my area.

☐ I would like an application form to study Eckankar further. Please send me more information about the twelve-month Eckankar study discourses on dreams.

Please type or print clearly   940

Name _____

Street _____ Apt. # _____

City _____ State/Prov. _____

Zip/Postal Code _____ Country _____

(Our policy: Your name and address are held in strict confidence. We do not rent or sell our mailing lists. Nor will anyone call on you. Our purpose is only to show people the ECK way home to God.)